I Can't Believe It's Yoga
for Kids!

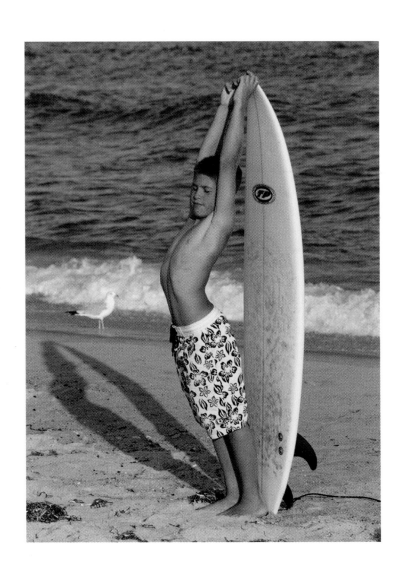

I Can't Believe It's
Yoga
for Kids!

Lisa Trivell

Photography by
Peter Field Peck

Hatherleigh Press
New York
A Getfitnow.com Book

Hatherleigh Press/GETFITNOW.com Books
An Affiliate of W.W. Norton & Company, Inc.
5-22 46th Avenue, Suite 200
Long Island City, NY 11101
1-800-367-2550

Visit our website: www.getfitnow.com

Disclaimer:

Before beginning any strenuous exercise program consult your physician. The
author and publisher of this book and workout disclaim any liability, personal or
professional, resulting from the misapplication of any of the training procedures
described in this publication.

All GETFITNOW.com titles are available for bulk purchase, special
promotions, and premiums. For more information, please contact the manager
of our Special Sales Department at 1-800-367-2550.

Library of Congress Cataloging-in-Publication Data
TO COME

Cover design by Lisa Fyfe
Text design and composition by Dede Cummings Designs

Photographed by Peter Field Peck
with Canon® cameras and lenses on Fuji® print film
Printed in Canada on acid-free paper
10 9 8 7 6 5 4 3 2 1

I would like to dedicate this book to my two children, Amanda and Dylan, whom I love so much.

Also to all the kids pictured in the book – thanks for your participation and inspiration. I hope this book reaches many children who can start to integrate yoga into their lives.

ACKNOWLEDGEMENTS

I would like to give special thanks to Tracy Tumminello for her continued support and editing talent. She has a great sense of humor and the kids really enjoyed working with her.

For Peter Field Peck, a very talented photographer, who has a special eye for capturing kids in motion having fun.

My publisher Andrew Flach, who had faith in this project from the beginning.

And Kevin Moran, Maria Rothwell, Fleur and Len Harlin for all their generosity and support.

Special thanks to all the children who have studied yoga with me and to the kids that worked so enthusiastically on the book: Max Baez, Susannah Edelbaum, Katherine Esposito, Michael Esposito, Kinara Flagg, Liz Dankowski, Betty Dankowski, Amanda Gang, Dylan Gang, Kevin Geiger, Chris Golden, Kimberly Havlik, Annie Lee, Celina Leroy, Caroline McCann, Jami Moore, Nicholas Moore, Conner Moran, Kevin Moran Jr., Nora Moran, Tom Moran, Chris Poli, Emma Poli, Michael Poli, and Dale Sprayregen.

CONTENTS

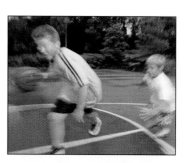

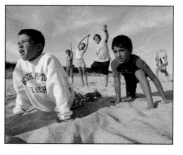

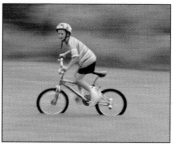

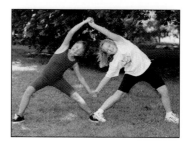

I Can't Believe It's Yoga for Kids!

PART I
INTRODUCTION

Life can be very busy for kids these days. I have two children ages 11 and 9, and I know how their days can be so hectic and sometimes stressful. It is important for children to learn stress reduction techniques early in their lives. Between schoolwork, after-school activities and hanging out with friends, it is easy to get overwhelmed. Children and adults both need to take the time to learn the skills of relaxation. Besides being a terrific stress-reducer, yoga is a great total body workout. It stretches and tones many unused muscle groups while incorporating breathing techniques.

Yoga gives children the time they need to slow down from their busy daily activities and a chance to progress with exercises at their own pace. As one of the few non-competitive sports, yoga teaches children how to improve their strength and flexibility through practice and patience. Children will find that by studying yoga and practicing a little each day, their flexibility will increase, helping to improve athletic performance and prevent injury.

There has been research showing a strong connection between yoga and cognitive learning in children. The breathing and centering exercises in yoga enhance concentration skills and improve patience. Furthermore, yoga promotes balance through the repetition of exercises on both sides of the body. In addition to balancing the muscles and nerves, this also helps balance the right and left sides of the brain. Using both sides of the brain helps integrate a child's creative and analytical faculties, improving his or her ability to learn on various levels. We all learn in different ways–spatially, visually, emotionally and analytically. Yoga helps us integrate and develop each of these areas of our brain.

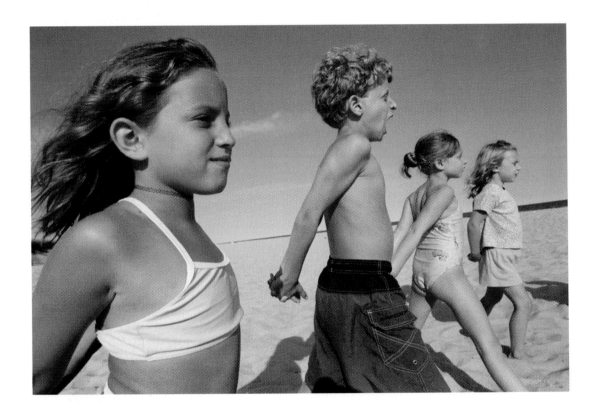

Another, and perhaps the most important, element of yoga is that it is fun to do. Yoga can be done alone, with a friend or in a group. Kids can do the exercises when they wake-up, to stretch before sports or to just unwind at the end of the day. Yoga exercises increase energy as they release tension. Helping children feel centered, yoga can improve memory and boost self-confidence.

Success in yoga is measured by a child's progress–how one's balance improves, how far one stretches, and what new muscles groups one notices. Children will be able to take this new awareness of their bodies and minds with them throughout their lives.

PART II
WHY WE DO YOGA

Yoga is a science of movement, originating thousands of years ago in India. Yogis would meditate in the woods and carefully observe the animals and birds around them. They would tune their bodies to become supple, strong and alert, mimicking the movements they observed in nature to create yoga postures. The yogis named exercises after animals, such as the cobra, cat and dog. Other exercises were named for their surroundings, such as mountain, tree and lotus.

The yogis found that yoga increased energy and concentration by integrating stretching and strengthening exercises with synchronized breathing. Yoga is a powerful system of body and mind exercises that anyone can do. It encourages us to understand how our bodies work and

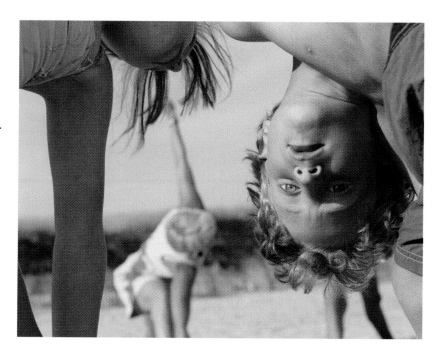

teaches us to focus from the inside out. Through exercises and conscious breath, yoga helps us get in touch with our personal energy.

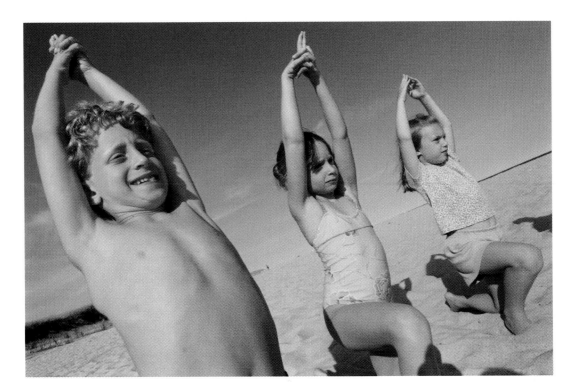

Posture

Yoga helps develop good posture by balancing muscle groups throughout the body. It makes children conscious of working three dimensionally–not thinking only straight ahead but becoming aware of the sides and the back of the body. Yoga creates an awareness of how the body moves and feels by concentrating on poses that awaken various muscle groups.

Yoga also helps posture by flexing and arching the back. It stretches the torso from side to side, gently twisting the spine from bottom to top in both directions. This movement strengthens the back muscles and lengthens the spine to increase kinetic awareness. Increased kinetic awareness enables a child to remember the sensation of correct posture and apply it throughout the day.

By sitting up tall with your shoulders down, back lengthened and neck free of tension, kids are going to feel more alert and awake. The combination of body awareness and balanced muscles is the key to improved posture.

How Yoga Improves Posture

- Teaches correct deep breathing to expand the chest.
- Increases awareness of tension in the shoulders and neck and how to release it.
- Uses the internal and external abdominal muscles to help you stand or sit up tall.
- Emphasizes bending and stretching from the hip sockets rather then the lower back, helping to lengthen the spine, instead of rounding it.
- Encourages resting on the sit bones rather then the lower spine, which also can round the back.

Self Esteem

Kids between the ages of 10 and 16 need to feel good about themselves. This is a time of substantial change in their lives, both emotionally and physically. Yoga can help smooth this transition by balancing the body, improving self-confidence and releasing stress.

As children and young adults feel more relaxed and aware of the connection between their body and mind, their self-image and confidence improves. *Good posture increases self-image, and feeling good about yourself improves posture.*

Peer Pressure

What is cool? Yoga is a growing trend in our popular culture today. Kids see music stars, actors and sports figures practicing yoga and reaping the benefits. Yoga helps the musician remain limber and stay centered while touring; helps the

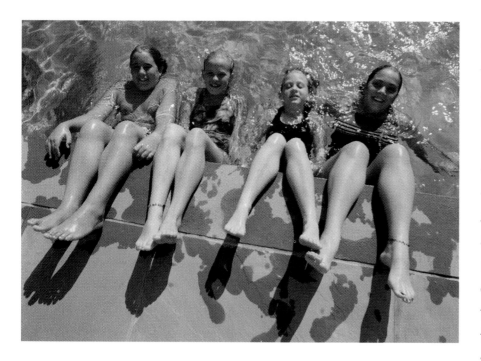

movie star by toning the muscles and reducing anxiety; and helps the professional athlete by increasing focus and enhancing flexibility. Adults, teenagers, and kids are now more curious than ever to experience the numerous benefits of practicing yoga. Yoga is an excellent opportunity for children to discover something new and share what they have learned with friends.

Anxiety

Yoga can help reduce performance anxiety before sports, tests and speeches. When children are in a music, theater or dance performance, they naturally experience jitters before show time. Knowing some of the basics of yoga will give them the tools to relax, center themselves and remember their lines. These days, when so much pressure is put on tests and more is demanded of kids academically, it is very important for children to learn stress management skills.

Growing Pains

As kids go through growth spurts during their childhood and adolescence, tendons and muscles can get very tight. Yoga helps stretch and loosen expanding muscles, helping to ease the discomfort of growing pains.

Appearance

Yoga can improve a child's complexion by balancing the glands, which regulate active hormones in pre-teens and teens. This can also help stabilize metabolism to regulate weight gain. Yoga exercises improve circulation, leading to healthier and clearer skin.

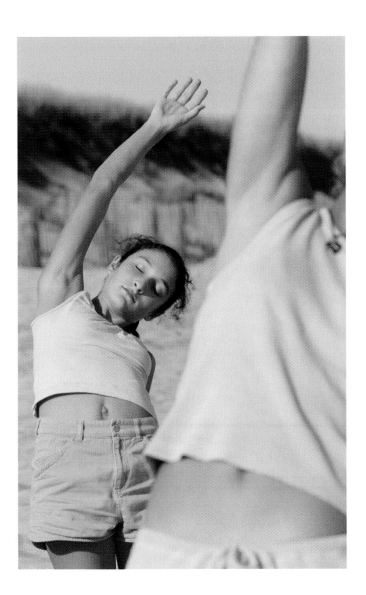

Benefits

- fun and creative
- teaches you exercises to do alone or in a group
- improves your flexibility
- improves body image
- increases self-confidence
- increases strength in both small and big muscle groups
- improves balance and agility
- teaches the connection between body and mind
- posture and muscle awareness
- balances the muscle groups
- enhances one's sensitivity, self-control and enjoyment in sharing

- improves athletic performance

- helps prevent injuries

- helps weight maintenance by regulating metabolism

- channels nervous energy

- helps develop self-discipline and poise

- fuels the imagination and enhances creativity

- releases tension and helps balance emotions

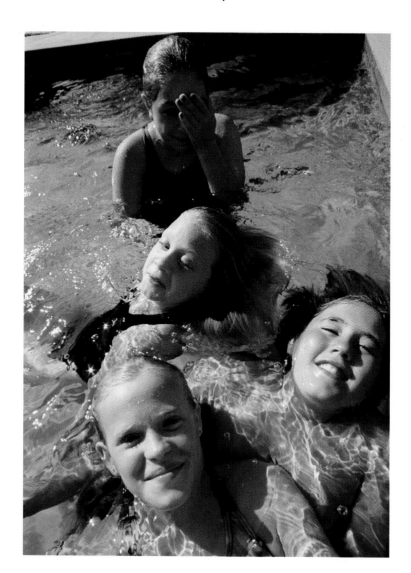

PART III
BREATHING

Breathing techniques are an important element of any yoga routine. Breathing exercises relax and invigorate as they help to center the mind. For example, a slow three-part breath can be used before and during a test or competition; fire breath is particularly beneficial in the morning or mid-afternoon when a child needs an energy boost; and punching bag breath is calming when a child feels angry or upset.

Before you begin your yoga routine, take a few minutes to focus your attention inward. Sit cross-legged and close your eyes. Feel your breath enter and exit through your nose to encourage full breathing. Envision the air passing through

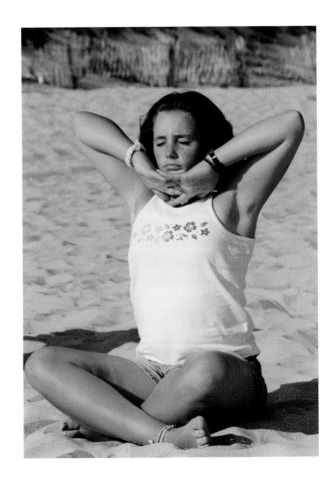

your nose and sinuses, and the diaphragm muscles under your ribcage dropping to allow the lower, middle and, then, upper lungs to fill. Picture your lungs three-dimensionally as two balloons expanding with clean, fresh air. Feel the warm air exit your lungs through your nose as you exhale, relaxing your muscles. Keep your chest lifted and lengthen your spine. Breathe in energy as you exhale tension.

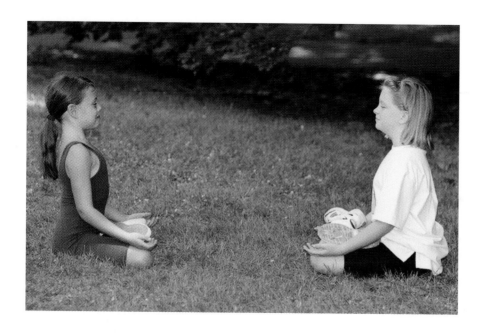

Our respiration and blood circulation work closely together to provide the constant supply of oxygen needed for our brain and muscles. We cannot live without oxygen, which is transferred to our bloodstream with each inhale. Our heart then pumps the blood to all areas of the body. After the blood is circulated throughout the body, it returns to the heart for oxygen. The heart pumps the blood through the lungs to restore its oxygen and circulates through the body again. This circulation process repeats itself over and over.

Do not be concerned if you have difficulty synchronizing your breathing with the exercises at first. The most important thing to remember is to not hold your breath, and to exhale completely while in each pose. The more you practice yoga, the more naturally correct breathing will come. Try to remember to inhale as you expand, exhale as you contract. It is important to breathe as you stretch because with each exhale, you can reach further into the stretch.

BREATHING EXERCISES

Three Part Breath – Visualize the shape of your lungs as they expand three-dimensionally from the front, back and sides. Relax the diaphragm muscle, which attaches at the bottom of the rib cage. Allow the lower, middle and upper sections of your lungs to fill as you inhale and count to three.

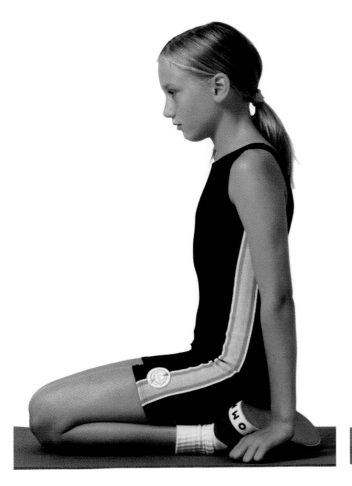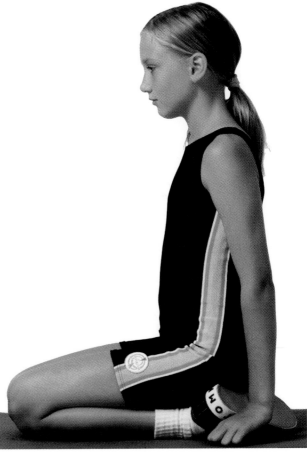

Three Part Breath

Angel Breath – Kneel or stand with your hands in front of your chest, and your palms together with your fingers interlaced. As you inhale, lift your elbows up and your head back. Then, exhale through your mouth, slowly bringing your elbows together and your head level.

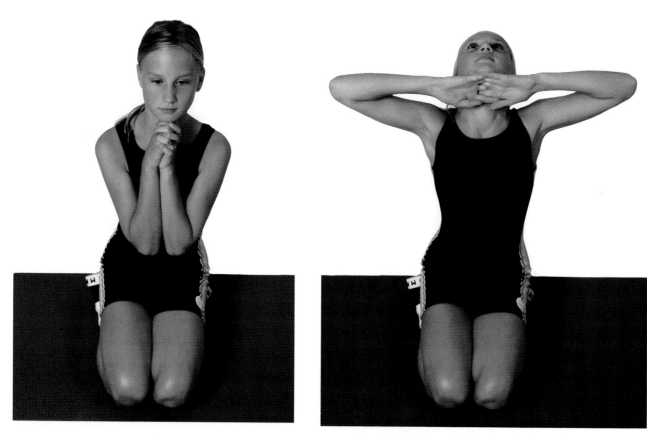

Angel Breath

Bunny Breath – On your knees with your hips resting on your heels, take two short inhales through your nose and a longer, fast exhale through the mouth.

Fire Breath – Sit cross-legged and concentrate on taking numerous quick, short breaths as you contract your stomach muscles as you exhale.

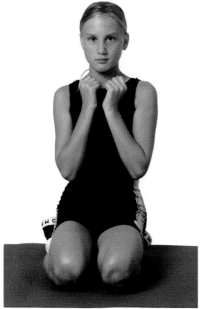

Energizer Punching Bag Breath – On your knees, make fists and breathe through your nose, exhaling as you punch in front of you.

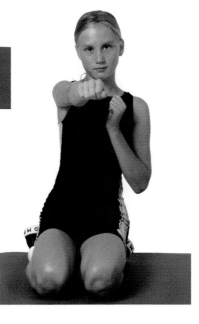

Energizer Punching Bag Breath

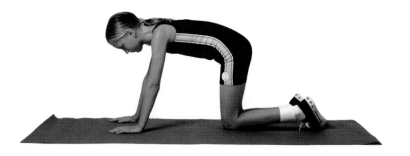

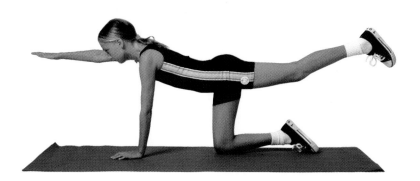

Table Breath – Kneeing on all fours, lift your right arm and left leg parallel to the ground and inhale. Exhale and return to the table position. Inhale and exhale through the nose as you quicken your breath and do a set of 10 on each side.

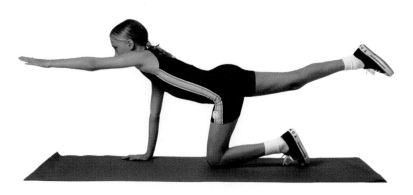

Table Breath

PART IV
EXERCISES

Yoga exercises require the involvement of both a person's body and the mind. The stretches and isometric strength training are challenging, yet safe, while the deep breathing calms your mind and refreshes your body. The following exercises can be done in the sequence that follows, or arranged into shorter 10 or 15 minute routines such as the ones listed in Part IX.

A few things to remember when doing yoga:

- Eat very lightly one hour before and after practicing yoga. Eat a larger meal two or more hours before doing yoga.

- Have as few distractions as possible around you to make it easier to concentrate (i.e. pets, parents, loud music).

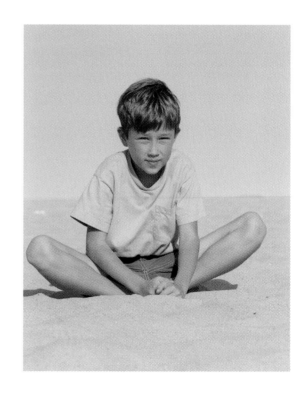

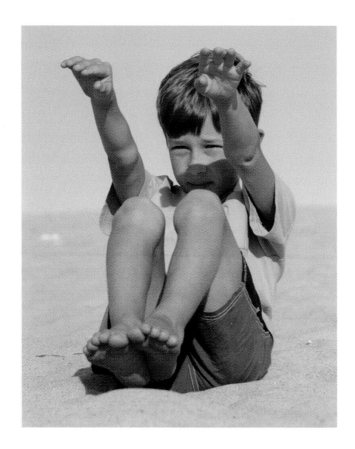

- Don't worry if you do not perform the exercise perfectly. As you continue to practice yoga, you gain more experience and can absorb more of the details.

- Perform the exercises slowly and attentively. Try to concentrate on the posture and what you are feeling.

- Never strain.

- Above all else, have fun!

Half Lotus – Sit cross-legged with one foot on top of the opposite thigh and the bottom of the foot turned up. With your back lengthened, keep your shoulders down and your neck long. Switch leg positions and repeat.

Benefit: adds flexibility to hips sockets.

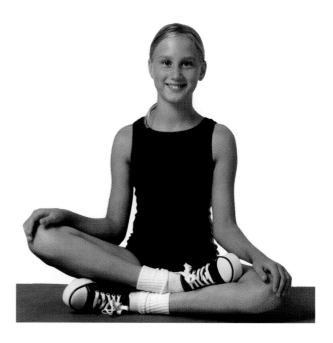

Half Lotus

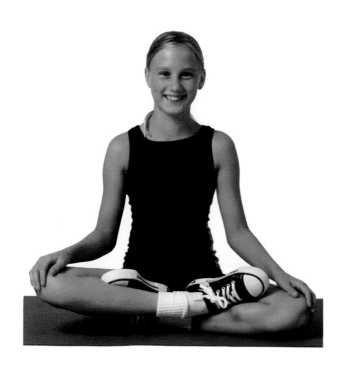

Full Lotus

Full Lotus – Sit in the same position as the half lotus, but cross both feet over the opposite thighs.

Benefit: encourages correct posture and increases concentration.

17

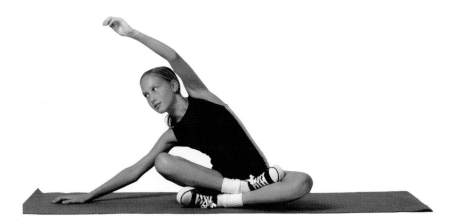

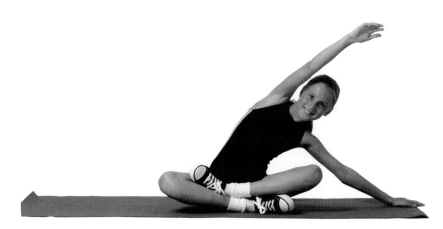

Seated Side Stretch

Seated Side Stretch – Sit in a comfortable cross-legged position. Drop your right hand to the floor beside you and stretch your left arm up and over your head close to your ear. Breathe in and out three times and repeat on the opposite side.

Benefit: tones the hips and torso, and encourages full breathing.

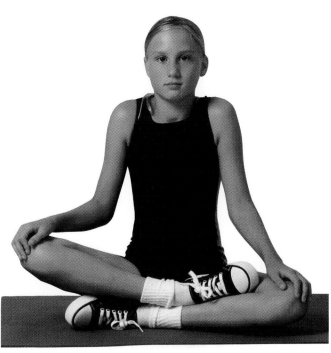

Shoulder Rolls

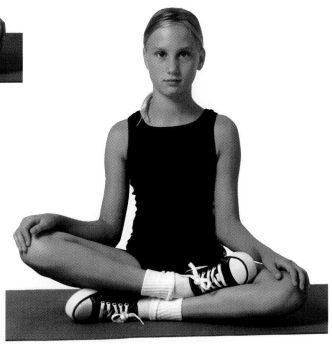

Shoulder Rolls – Roll your shoulders forward, up to your ears, back to your shoulder blades, and down. Repeat five times.

Benefit: relaxes and tones shoulder and neck muscles.

Neck rolls – Stretch your right ear to your right shoulder, bring your chin to chest, and stretch your left ear to left shoulder. Reverse directions and repeat three times.

Benefit: releases tension in the sides and back of the neck and jaw.

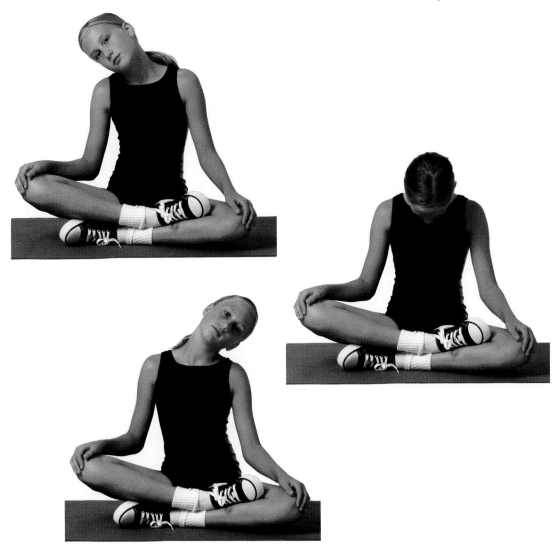

Neck rolls

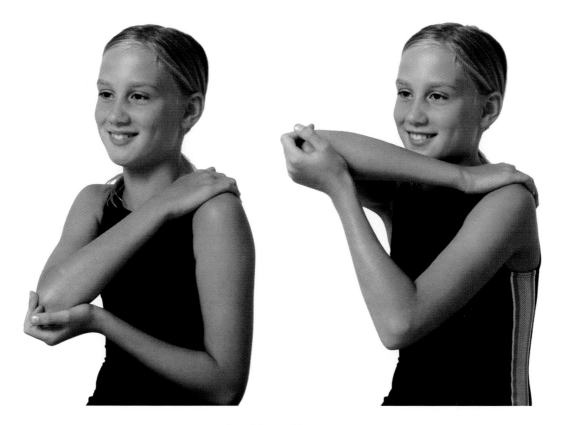

Shoulder Self-Massage

Shoulder Self-Massage – While sitting up straight in a chair or cross-legged on the floor, take your right hand and reach over to your left shoulder. Squeeze your left shoulder with your right hand. Then, take your fingertips and rub a little deeper in small circles using more pressure. Try to locate and release tightness in your muscles as you take deep full breaths. Repeat on the other shoulder.

Benefit: enables you think more clearly and to release stress in your shoulders, a common place for stored tension.

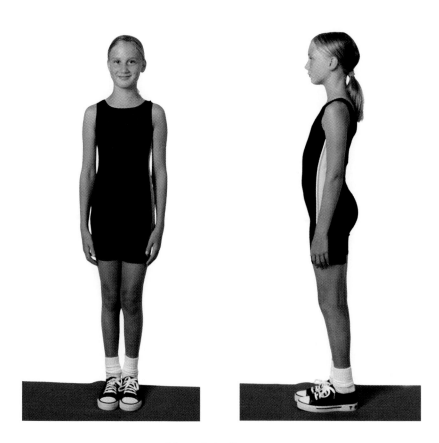

Mountain Pose

Mountain Pose – Stand up straight with your feet together. Stack your body so your knees are over your ankles, your hips are over your knees, and your ribcage is over your hips. Lengthen your neck so your jaw is parallel to the ground.

Benefit: increases awareness of your posture and is a good transition pose.

Forward Bend - From the mountain pose, slowly roll down one vertebra at a time until you are bending from the hip sockets. Feel your back and neck relax and let your arms dangle to your fingertips. Bend and straighten each leg.

Benefit: relaxes the back muscles and begins to stretch the hamstrings.

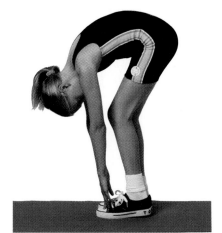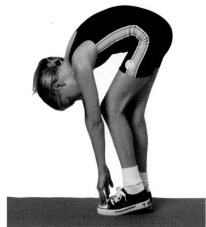

Forward Bend

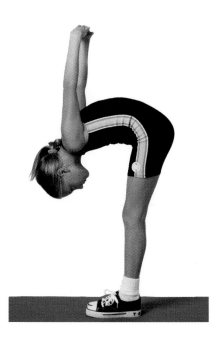

Swimmer's Stretch – With your feet together or hips-width apart, interlace your fingers behind you and slowly roll down the back. Allow your head to drop as you keep your arms straight.

Benefit: stretches the entire back of the body as well as all the shoulder muscles.

Swimmer's Stretch

23

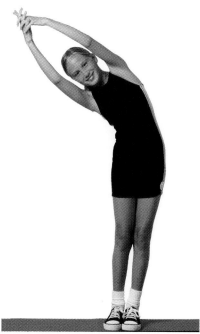

Half Moon

Half Moon – With your feet together, interlace your hands above your head, keeping your rib cage over your hips. Stretch your arms to the right as you stretch your hips to the left and switch side. Breathe in and out and repeat three times on both sides.

Benefit: tones the waist and encourages good posture and correct full breathing.

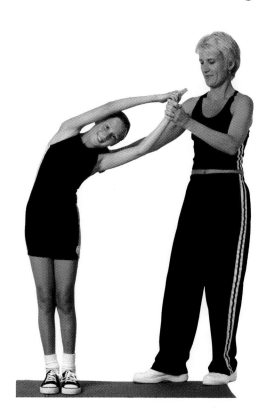

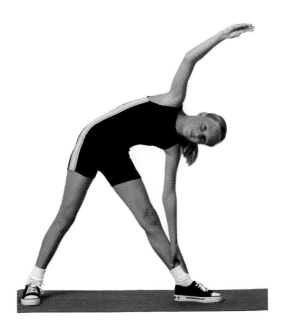

Triangle Side Stretch

Triangle Side Stretch – Stand with your feet more than shoulder-width apart, your right foot facing forward, and your left foot turned out. Line up the heel of your left foot with the arch of your right foot. Equally balance between both feet. Stretch your arms out to the sides parallel to the ground. Stretch your left hand down to your left shin and reach your right arm over your head close to your ear. Breathe fully three times and repeat on the other side.

Benefit: tones the waist and hips, improves posture and releases tension in the spine.

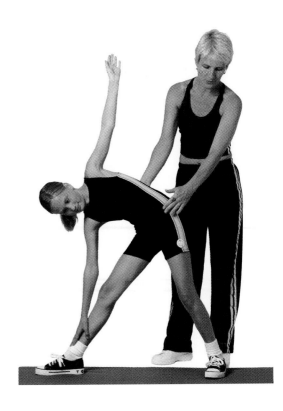

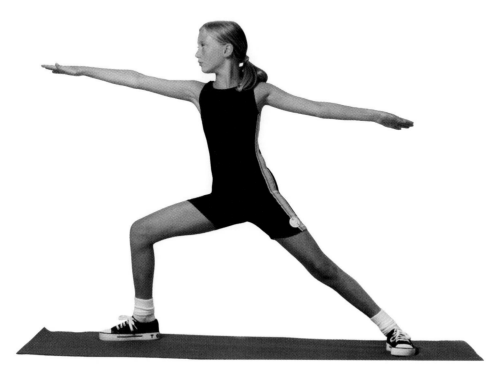

Warrior

Warrior – Starting in the same position as the triangle pose, bend your left knee over your left foot. Work toward having your left thigh parallel to the floor. Hold your arms out to the sides and gaze over your left fingertips.

Benefit: increases circulation and strengthens the thighs, lower back and stomach muscles.

Triangle Spinal Twist – Start from the triangle pose with your arms out to the sides, parallel to the floor. Reach your right arm to your left shin, and your left arm behind you up to the sky. Keep your back lengthened from the tailbone through the neck as you look behind you or up to your arm. Breathe in and out three times and reverse sides.

Benefit: balances the nervous system, and the muscles up and down the spine.

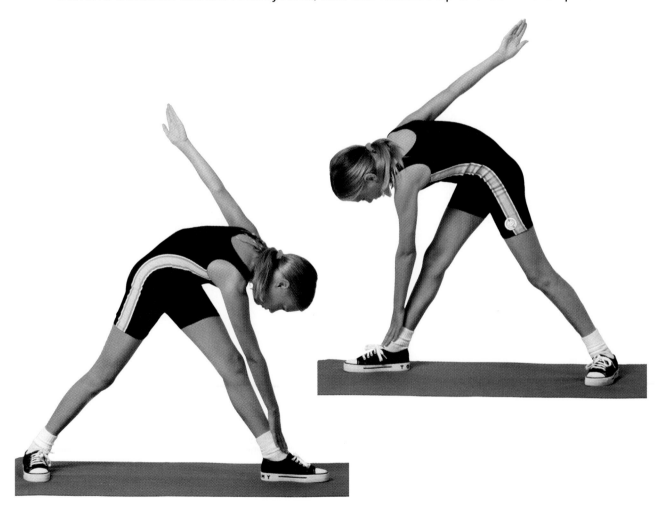

Triangle Spinal Twist

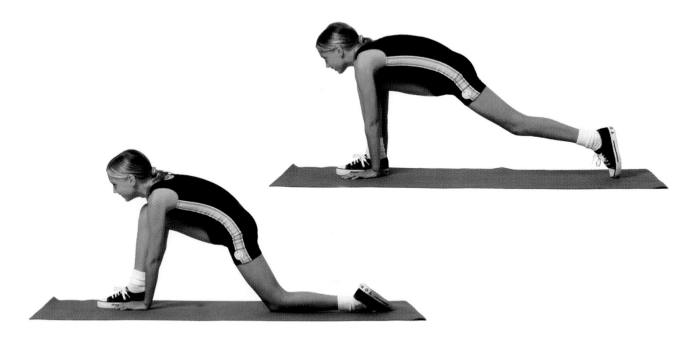

Lunges

Lunges – Start in the mountain pose and drop your right leg behind you as far as possible. Keep both hands on the ground for support as you bend and straighten your left leg three times. The last time you straighten your leg, hold the pose to feel the stretch. Repeat with opposite leg.

Benefit: this is a wonderful stretch for the quadriceps, and it improves flexibility for many sports.

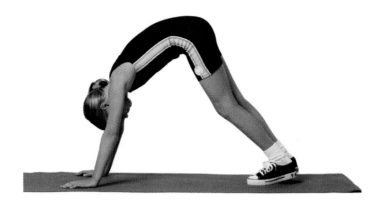

Down Dog

Down Dog – Press your feet and hands into the floor as you lift your hips up in the air. Concentrate on lengthening the back muscles and stretching your hamstrings. Bend and straighten your legs slowly for a deeper stretch. Take three full breaths.

Benefit: strengthens the back muscles, releases tension and activates the leg muscles.

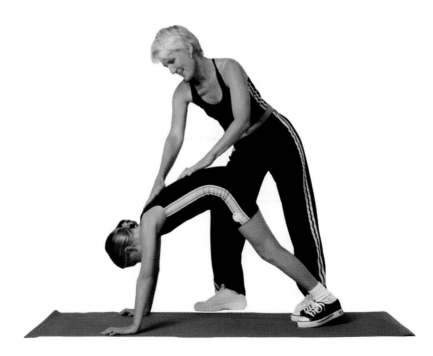

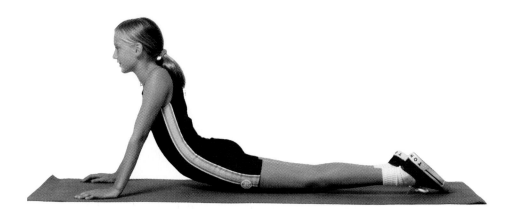

Up Dog

Up Dog – From the down dog position, drop your pelvis to the floor and arch your back. Tighten your hip muscles as you lift your chest off the floor.

Benefit: strengthens the lower back and tones the stomach muscles.

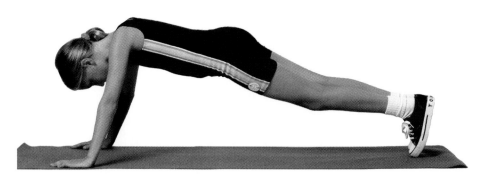

Plank

Plank – Resting on your hands and the balls of your feet, level your body so that your back and legs are straight. Tighten your buttocks and use your arm muscles to maintain the position.

Benefit: strengthens the upper back, arms and stomach muscles.

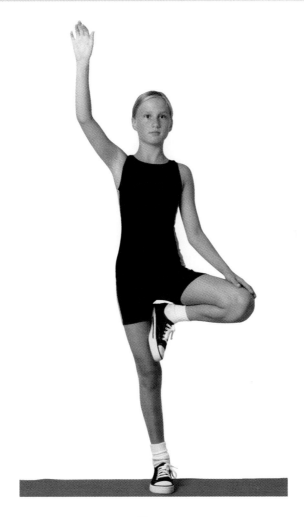

Tree

Tree – Balance on your left foot and bend your right leg, resting your right foot on your left inner thigh. Reach arms up over your head with your palms together. Focus on a stationary point in front of you to keep your balance.

Benefit: improves balance and concentration.

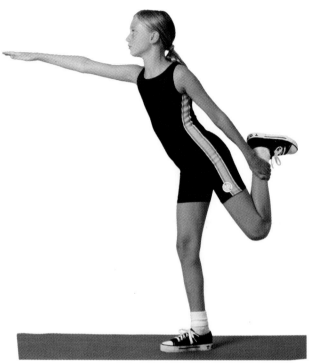

Dancer

Dancer – Stand with your feet a few inches apart. Shift your weight onto your right leg as you hold your left foot behind you with your left hand. Focus on a stationary point and pay attention to your breathing to help you balance. Raise your right arm over your head as you stretch your left knee and foot backward. Breathe and repeat on the opposite side.

Benefit: stretches your thigh muscles and quadriceps; and improves balance, coordination and vitality.

Flamingo – Balancing on your left leg, stretch your arms out to the sides and extend your right leg behind you. Aim to bring your torso and right leg parallel to the ground. Focus on a stationary point in front of you.

Benefit: helps to focus the mind and increase agility.

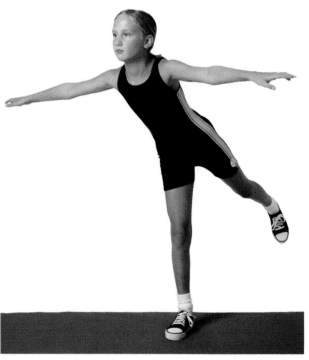

Flamingo

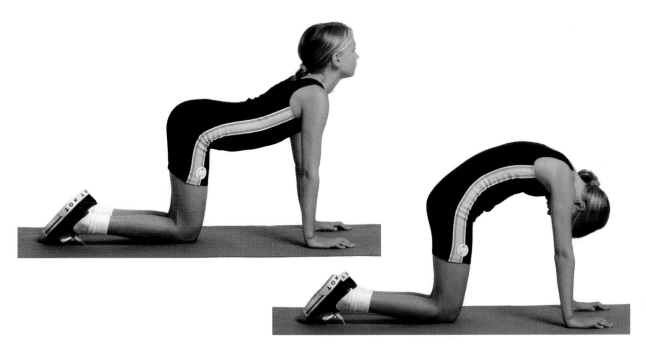

Cat

Cat – On your hands and knees, lengthen your back from the tailbone through the neck. Inhale as you arch your back, and exhale as you round it. Repeat five times.

Benefit: releases tension in the back and helps to balance the nervous system.

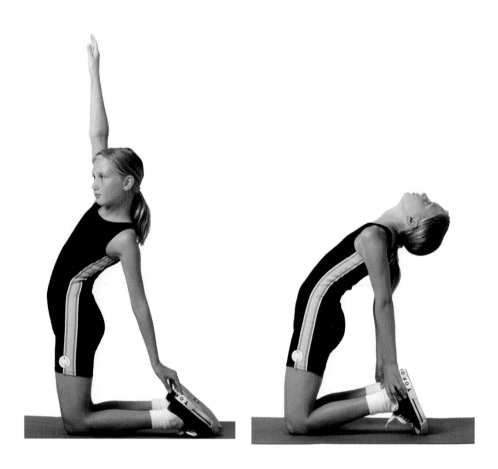

Camel

Camel – Kneel down with your legs shoulder-width apart. Slowly place your right hand on your right heel and your left hand on your left heel. As you arch your back, imagine the curve of your body is the shape of a camel's hump. Stay in the pose for a count of ten. Remember to breathe slowly and smoothly.

Benefit: strengthens the back; tones the hips and thigh muscles; trims the waist; increases flexibility in the spine; and keeps the stomach and bladder healthy by increasing circulation and toning surrounding muscles to improve digestion.

Child Pose – Starting on your knees, release your pelvis and sit on your heels. Lower your chest to your knees and stretch your arms out on the floor in front of you or down to your sides.

Benefit: a great restorative pose to release and re-energize your back.

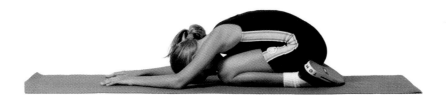

Child Pose

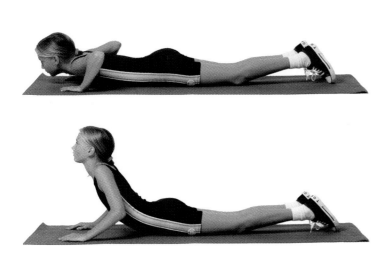

Cobra

Cobra – Lie on your stomach with your arms resting at your sides. Breathe slowly and smoothly. With your chin on the mat and your hands under your shoulders, use your back muscles to lift your chest off the ground. Press your hands slightly into the ground as you keep your hips and legs on the floor. Slowly lower your chest and relax your head to the side.

Benefit: helps keep the spine flexible and healthy; strengthens the shoulders, elbows and wrists; and increases circulation into the digestive tract.

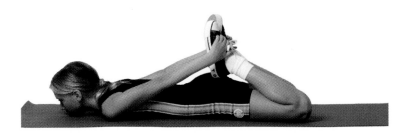

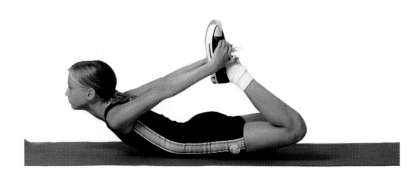

Bow

Bow – Lie on your stomach with your legs slightly apart and arms by your sides. Bend your knees and lengthen your chest as you reach back to hold your ankles. Slowly tilt your head back and pull your feet upward. Gently rock back and forth as you breathe smoothly. Stay in the pose as long as you can, then release your arms and legs back down to the floor.

Benefit: strengthens the back muscles, increases flexibility and expands your chest to help you to breathe more deeply.

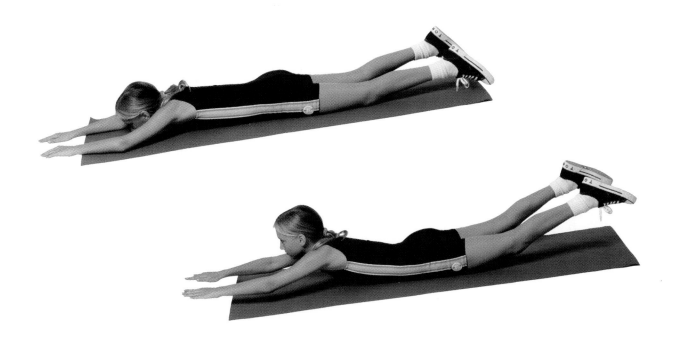

Superman

Superman – Lie on your stomach with your arms out in front of you and your chin resting on the mat. Exhale as you raise your chin, arms and legs up off the floor. Take three full breaths and relax your legs and arms. Repeat once.

Benefit: strengthens and balances the back muscles, and tones the stomach muscles.

Hurdler – Resting on your sit bones, the bottom of your hip girdle, keep your left leg straight and place your right foot against the inside of your left thigh. Be sure your left knee is facing up. Raise both arms above your head, interlace your fingers, and stretch your torso over your left leg. Reach forward to your toes for a count of three breaths, trying to stretch further with each exhale. Repeat with the opposite leg.

Benefit: lengthens the hamstring muscles and releases tightness in the back and hips.

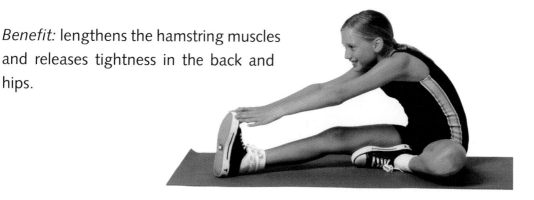

Hurdler

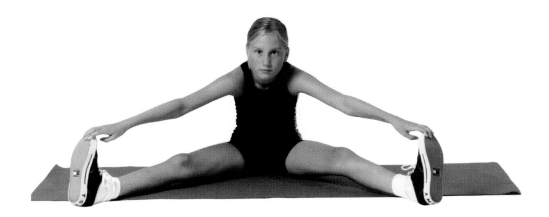

Straddle

Straddle – Rest on your sit bones with your legs as far apart as you can stretch. Lift your chest and reach your arms out on the floor in front of you or to your toes. Take three full breaths, stretching further with each exhale.

Benefit: opens the hip sockets to stretch the back and hamstrings, and stretches and tones the inner thigh muscles.

Boat – Balance on your sit bones as you extend your legs and arms out in front of you. Start with your knees slightly bent and work toward straightening your legs. Continue to breathe smoothly and relax your neck muscles.

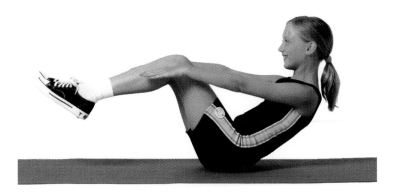

Boat

Benefit: tones abdominal muscles, transverse and oblique.

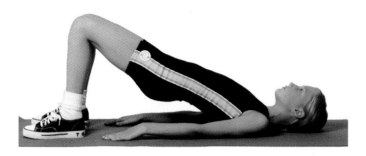

Half Bridge

Half Bridge – Lie on your back with your knees bent. Start by relaxing your back and neck into the ground and slowly lift your pelvis one vertebra at a time until you feel the weight across your shoulders. Interlace the fingers under your hips and tighten your buttocks . Hold the pose for a count of three breaths and slowly relax back down to the ground.

Benefit: increases circulation and awareness in the back, improves posture, and balances the nervous system.

Bridge – Start in the same position as the half bridge. Place your hands on the ground above your shoulders with your fingers facing you. As you exhale, push up off your hands and feet to arch your body. Hold for a count of ten breaths and slowly return back to the floor.

Benefit: a wonderful exercise for the back and stomach.

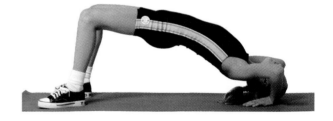

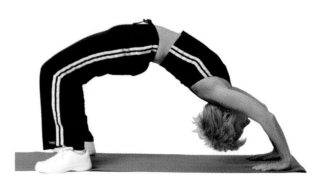

Bridge

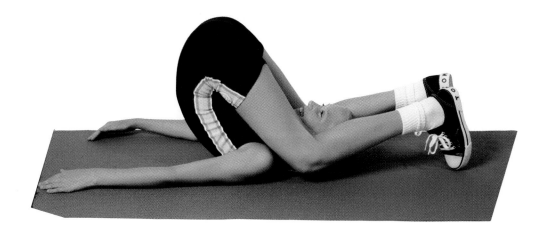

Plow

Plow – Lie on your back and bend your knees. Roll back until your knees are over your head by your ears. Relax in this position with your head facing straight up to keep the neck aligned. Support your back with your hands and breathe smoothly. Either straighten your legs into the shoulder stand or roll down into a half bridge.

Benefit: excellent exercise for overall health, increases circulation to the skin and hair, and releases tightness in the shoulders.

Shoulder Stand – From the plow position, slowly straighten one leg up at a time until both feet are pointing upward. Gradually move your hands up your back until your body is as straight as you can hold it comfortably. Breathe smoothly and hold this position for as long as it is comfortable. Slowly lower your legs into the plow position and use your stomach muscles to roll your legs back to the ground.

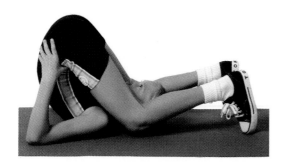

Benefit: stretches the entire body and is good for balancing the thyroid gland.

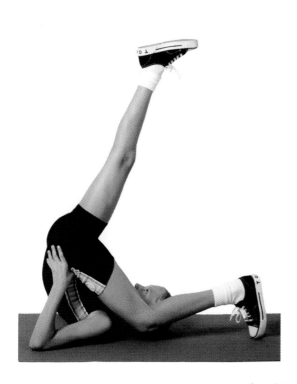
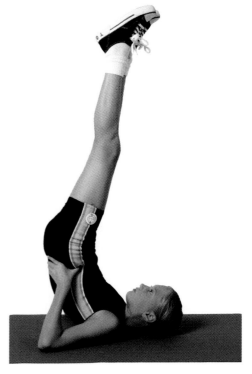

Shoulder Stand

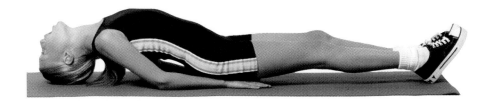

Fish

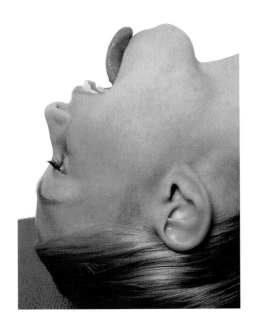

Fish – Lying on your back, arch your body from your lower back to your head. Use your back muscles to balance gently on your elbows. Stick your tongue out.

Benefit: counterbalances the shoulder stand.

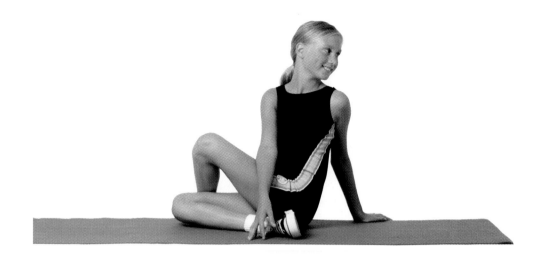

Seated Spinal Twist

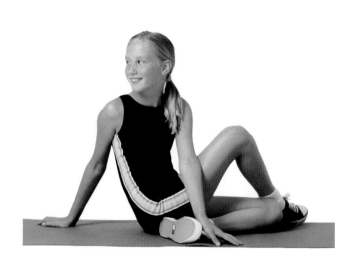

Seated Spinal Twist – Sit with your legs stretched out in front of you and bend your right leg over your left leg. Bend your left leg into your right hip. Reach your right arm behind you and press your left arm gently against the inside of your right thigh. Stretch your chin toward your right shoulder as you take three full breaths. Each time you inhale, lengthen your spine, and twist further on each exhale. Slowly untwist in the opposite direction. Come back to center and repeat.

Benefit: releases tension in the back, balances the spine and helps you to think more clearly.

EYE RELAXATION EXERCISES

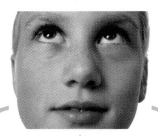

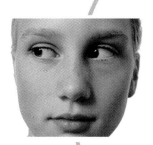

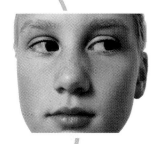

Clock – Sit or stand tall as you breathe slowly and smoothly. Imagine there is a big clock in front of you. Without your head moving, look up at 12, over to 3, down to 6, and over to 9, holding each for ten seconds. Then, roll your eyes clockwise three times. Stop and take three long breaths before rolling your eyes counter-clockwise three times.

Benefit: strengthens the eye muscles and relieves tension that can occur from reading, studying or staring at a computer screen.

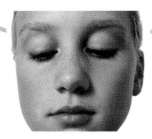

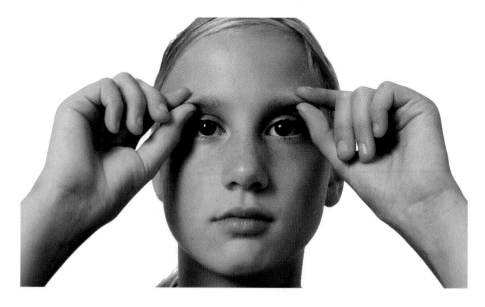

Brow Pinch

Brow Pinch – Find the ridge of the forehead above the eyes. Place your thumbs under the ridge and your index finger above it. Gently squeeze your eyebrows from the center out. Do both eyes at the same time and repeat three times.

Benefit: feels good, releases tension in the head and alleviates headaches and tired eyes.

Eye Rub – If you wear contact lenses, make sure you take them out before doing this exercise. Shake your hands out to release any tightness in them. With the index fingers, start at the corner of the eye and make tiny circles very lightly on your eyelids. Repeat in the center and to the outer corner.

Benefit: relieves eyestrain after reading or concentrating visually.

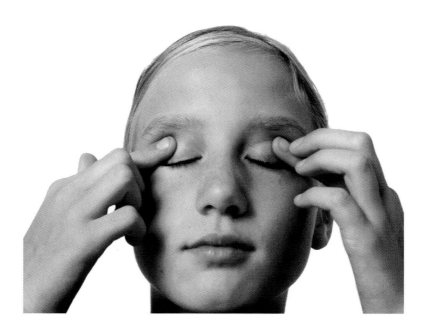

PART V
YOGA AND SPORTS

Yoga can also be a valuable addition to any pre- or post-sport stretching routine. It encourages complete range of motion while teaching kids how to stretch properly to improve athletic performance. If muscles, tendons and ligaments are lengthened and stretched properly, the potential for injury is significantly lowered. For sports such as baseball and hockey, yoga stretches can help balance muscle groups to increase coordination;

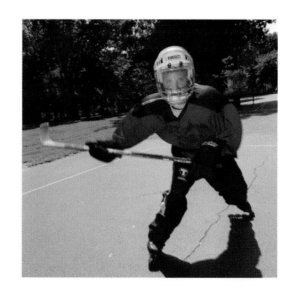

for tennis, yoga can improve agility; and for dance, yoga can be used to warm up and cool down before workouts.

Breathing

Yoga emphasizes tuning in to specific muscle groups as you stretch. The skill of concentration is essential to playing any sport well. The breathing techniques learned in yoga can be used to help children relax and focus on the game. These breathing exercises are also beneficial to aerobic endurance. Yoga helps us use our full lung capacity to improve our stamina.

Visualization

Before getting on the field or in the ring, after warming up, or on the night of a big game, practice a brief sports visualization exercise. Take three long breaths and roll your shoulders three times. Do three neck rolls in each direction as you massage the palms of your hands. Relax, close your eyes and picture yourself playing the sport with ease. If there's a particular move or play that you would like improve, picture it in your mind's eye. Feel the enjoyment that you get from playing the sport. This visualization can help relieve anxiety and improve confidence.

Improvement

At the end of a game, remember that it is not as important that you have won as it is that you have played well and to the best of your abilities. It is great to realize that you have improved your athletic ability. That is the essence of what

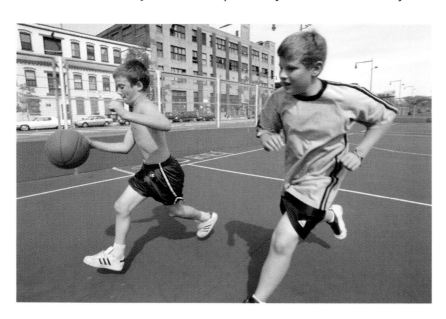

yoga teaches us—to work from the inside out to enhance flexibility and strength. If you are involved in team sports, encourage your teammates to practice these stretches and breathing techniques before the game, instead of sitting on the bench.

Even though yoga itself is non-competitive, it can greatly enhance athletic performance. Listed are a few sports-specific yoga exercises to stretch and strengthen various muscle groups:

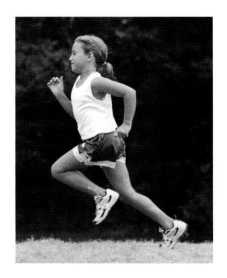 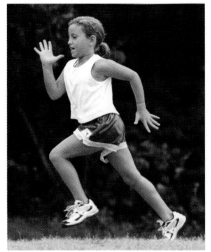 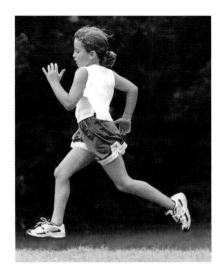

Running

- Lunge
- Dancer
- Hurdler

- **Sprinter's Lunge** – With your legs about three feet apart with one foot in front of the other, try to keep your back leg straight as you flex and release your front foot three times.

  Benefit: great stretch for the hamstrings and the calf muscles.

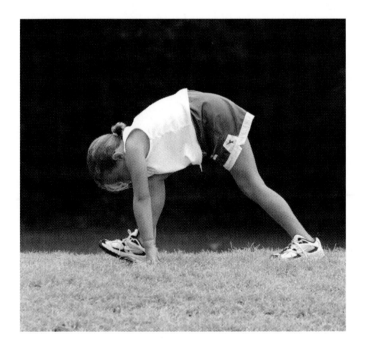

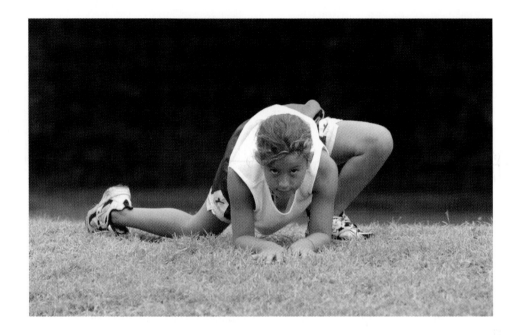

- **Side Lunge** – Lunge and stretch to the inside of your right foot as you rest your elbows on the ground.

  Benefit: releases tightness from the lower back, stretches the upper hamstrings and quadriceps.

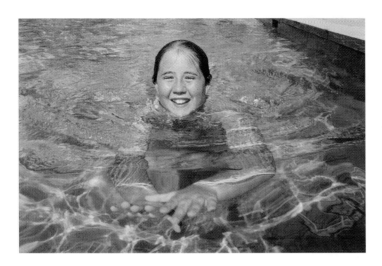

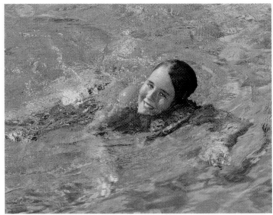

Swimming

- Warrior
- Swimmer's Stretch
- Plow

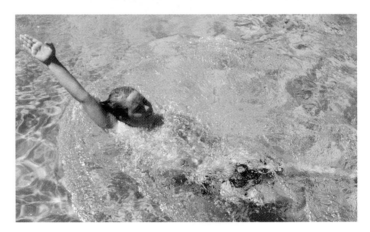

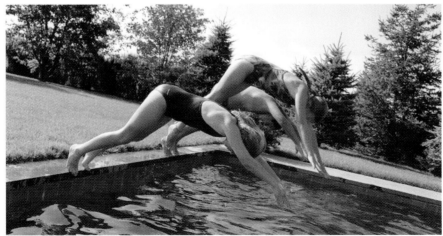

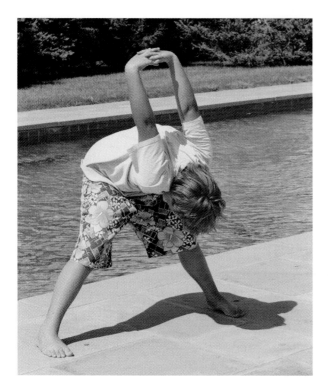

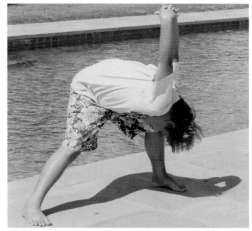

• **Swimmer's Stretch Variation** – Standing with your legs more than shoulder-width apart, interlace the fingers behind you and roll forward, one vertebra at a time. Use your arms to increase this stretch as you lunge from one leg to the other.

Benefit: great overall stretch for the back, lats and upper arm muscles.

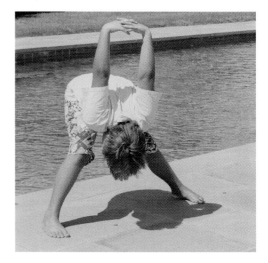

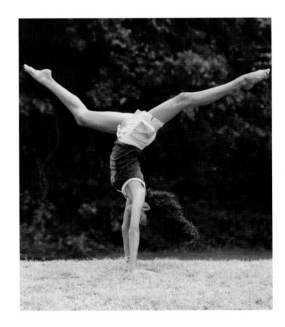

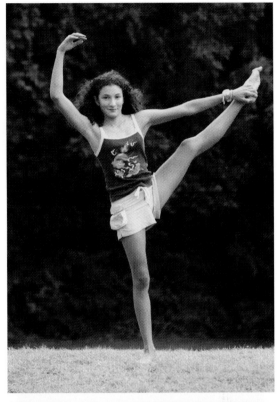

Gymnastics

- Seated spinal twist
- Cobra
- Plow
- Shoulder Stand
- Bridge

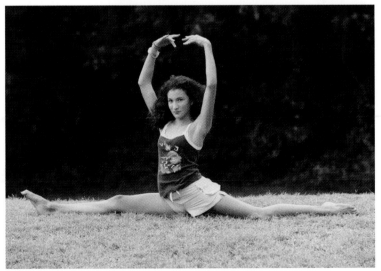

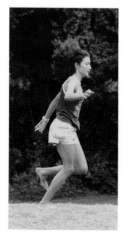 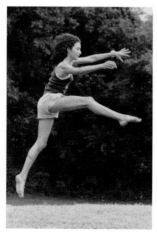 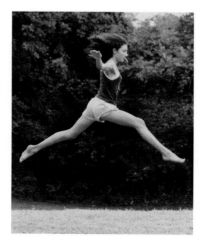 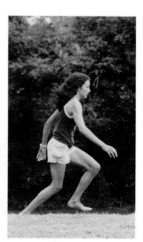

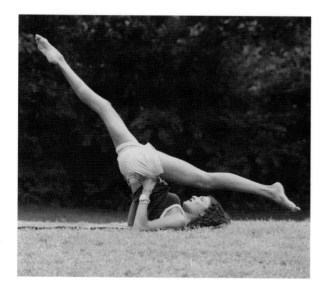

- **Shoulder Stand Variation** – Once you are in the shoulder stand, reach one leg forward and one leg back. Then, reverse legs and repeat.

  Benefit: stretches all the leg muscles.

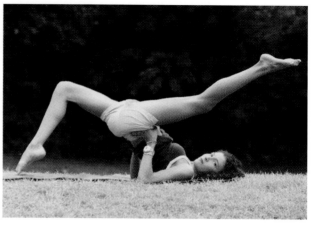

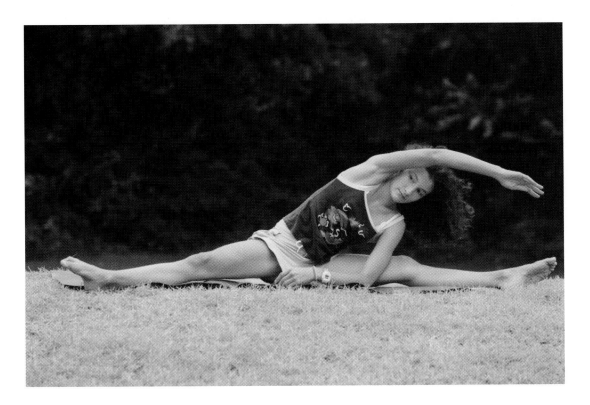

- **Side Straddle** – From the straddle pose, place your right hand or forearm on the ground near your knee. Lift your left arm up and over your head. Hold the pose for three breaths and repeat on the other side.

Benefit: stretches and tones the torso and stomach.

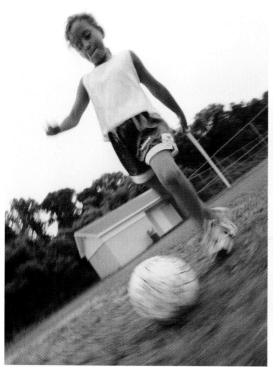

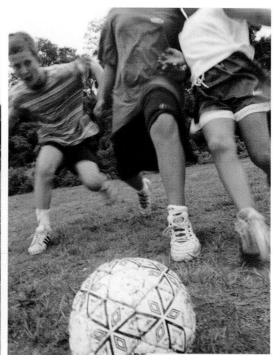

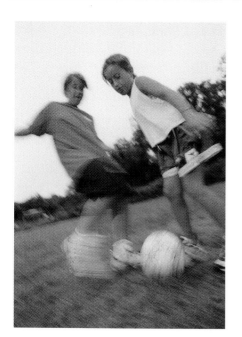

Soccer

- Straddle
- Hurdler
- Lunge
- Warrior

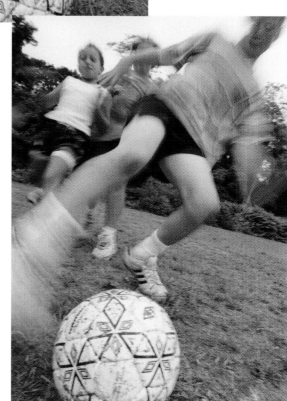

• **Butterfly** – Sit down with the soles of your feet together. Your pinky toes should be touching and your big toes should be spread apart. Breathe deeply on each exhale as you reach your chin and chest toward your feet.

Benefit: helps to identify and stretch your hip sockets, and is a great warm-up.

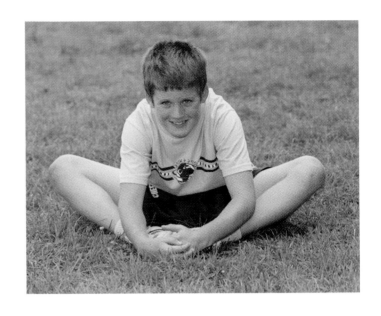

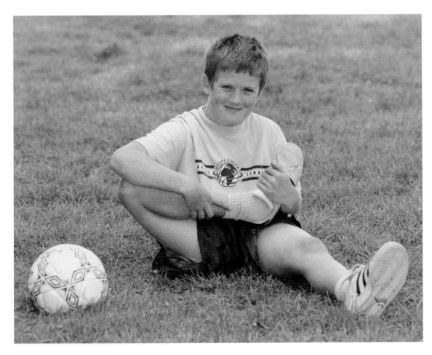

• **Rock-the-baby** – Sit in the cross-legged position and pick up your right leg. Hold and rock your leg gently from side to side.

Benefit: stretches the hips, releases the lower back and stretches the outer thigh.

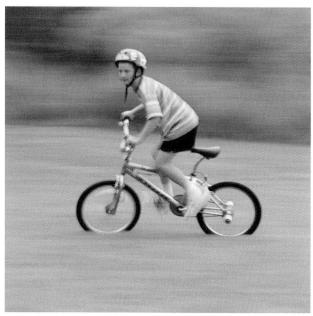

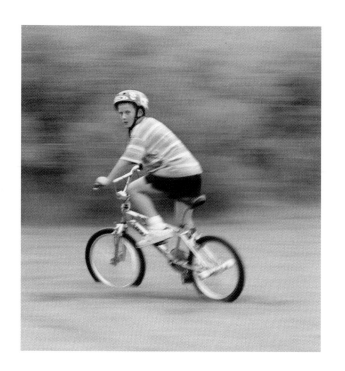

Biking

- Dancer
- Hurdler
- Forward Bend
- Lunge
- Swimmer's Stretch

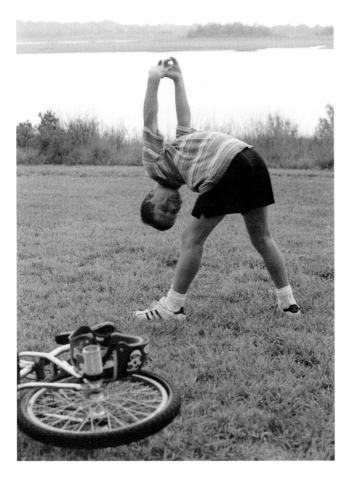

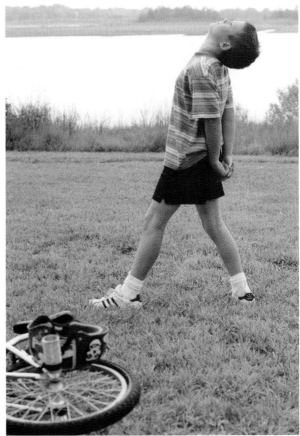

- **Hybrid Stretch** – Stand in the triangle pose with your right leg turned out and your left leg pointing forward. Interlace your fingers behind your back and roll your head down to your right knee. Breathe three times slowly and roll up.

  Benefit: stretches the entire back of the body.

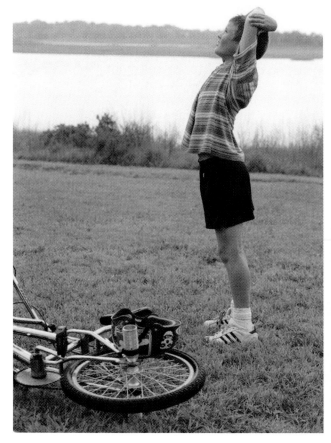

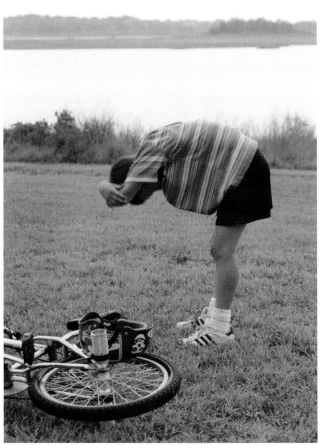

- **Mountain Bike Stretch** – Stand in the mountain pose, reach your arms over your head and hold your elbows. Tighten your hips, lift your chest and arch your upper back as you inhale. As you exhale, slowly roll forward. Take a full breath in and out before slowly rolling back up.

Benefit: releases tightness in the back and hamstrings, and is good for stretching the back and shoulder muscles.

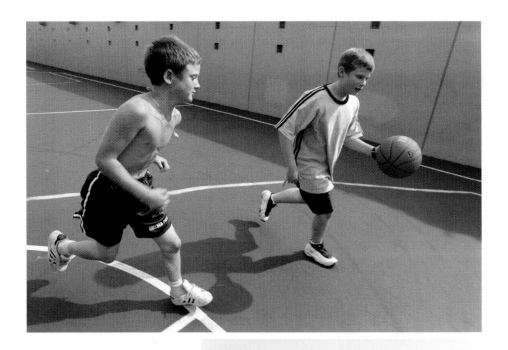

Basketball

- Hurdler
- Down Dog
- Plank Pose
- Up Dog

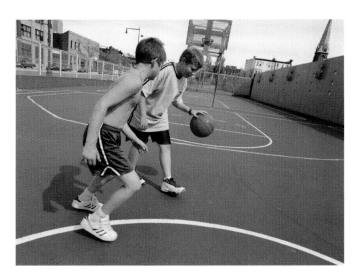

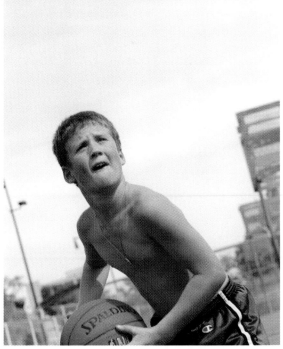

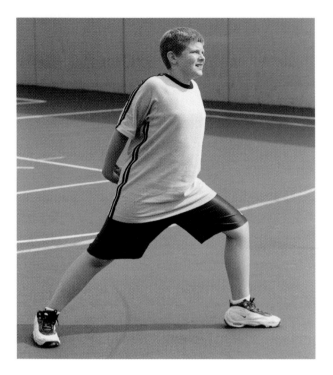

- **Warrior Back Stretch** – Start in the warrior pose and interlace your fingers behind you. Arch your back and feel the stretch across the front of your chest.

  Benefit: stretches the chest muscles, strengthens the leg muscles and encourages proper breathing.

- **Hoop Lunge** – With your feet three to four feet apart, bend your right knee and reach to your right foot. Take a deep breath and repeat on the opposite side.

  Benefit: loosens the hips and lower back.

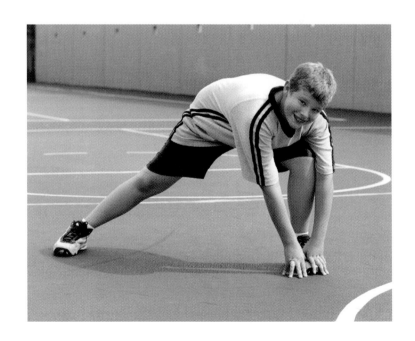

Baseball

- Triangle
- Triangle Spinal Twist
- Half Moon
- Plow

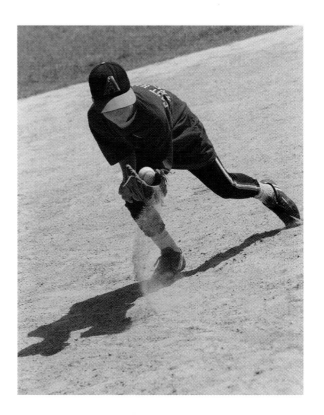

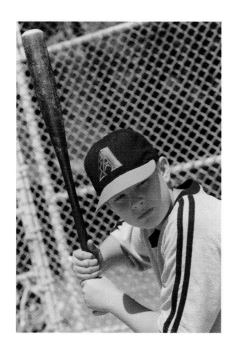

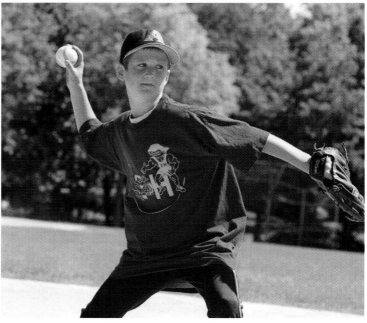

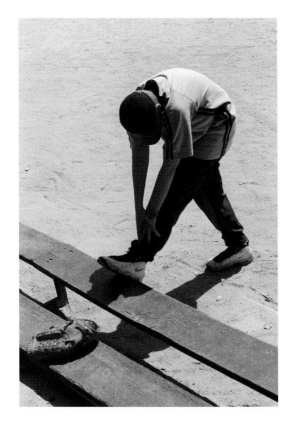

- **Bench Stretch** – With your right leg up on a bench or the bleachers, reach one arm up and over your head as you inhale. On the exhale, stretch forward and reach to your toes.

  Benefit: great for stretching the hamstrings and the back.

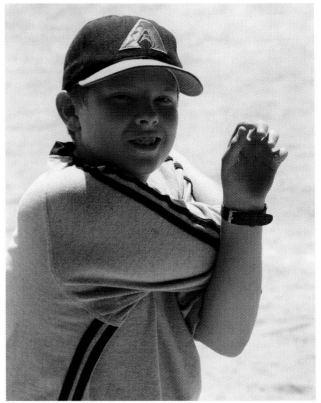

- **Hitter's Stretch** – Stretch your right arm across your chest and gently pull your right arm toward you with your left hand. Switch arms and repeat.

  Benefit: stretches the deltoid and rotator muscles.

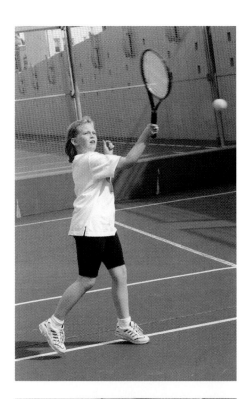

Tennis

- Lotus
- Shoulder Rolls
- Forward Bend
- Swimmer Stretch

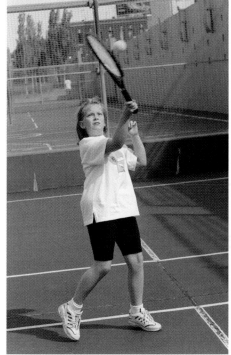

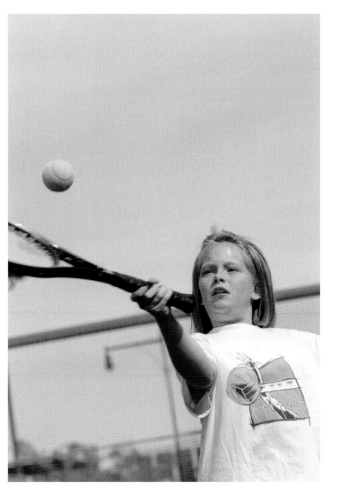

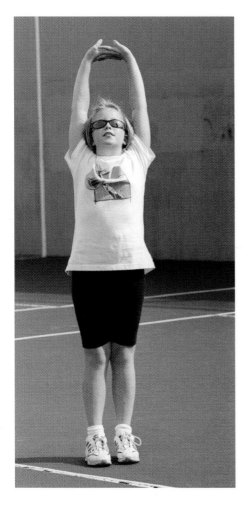

- **Half Moon Arch** – Interlace your hands over your head with your palms facing the sky. Plant your feet, lift your tummy and chest, and arch your upper and mid-back.

  Benefit: releases tension between the shoulder blades and stretches the muscles throughout the arms.

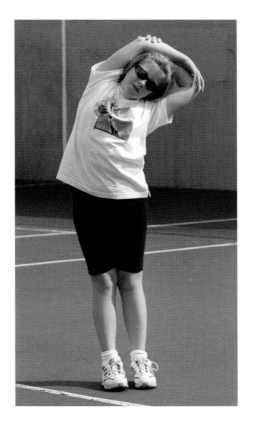

- **Elbow Hold Stretch** – Stand in the mountain pose, reach your arms over your head and hold your elbows. Stretch your arms to the left and your hips to the right. Take a full breath and repeat on opposite side.

  Benefit: stretches the shoulders and upper back.

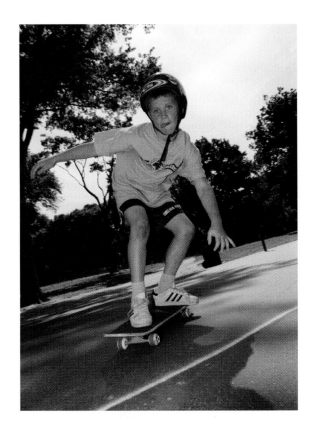 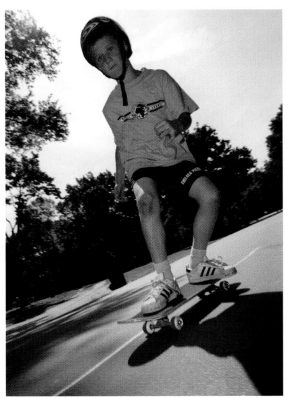

Skateboarding

- Tree Pose
- Bridge
- Plow
- Forward Fold

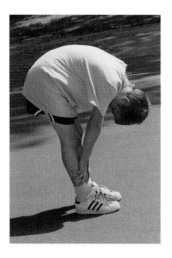

- **Half Pipe Bend** – With your feet hips-width apart, slowly roll down your back one vertebra at a time until your fingers reach your shins, ankles or toes, depending on your flexibility. Slowly roll back up.

  Benefit: releases stress along the entire spine and stretches the hamstrings.

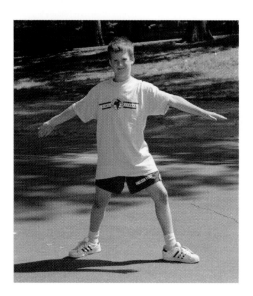 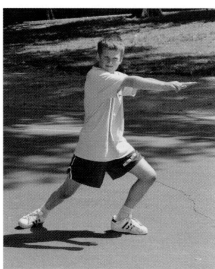

- **Bow & Arrow** – Start in the warrior pose with your feet three to four feet apart and your left leg turned out. Hold your arms out to the sides and keep your legs straight. As you exhale, bend your left knee and bring your right hand together with your left hand. Bend your right elbow as you pull your right arm back across your chest. Repeat three times on each side.

  Benefit: increases coordination and balance.

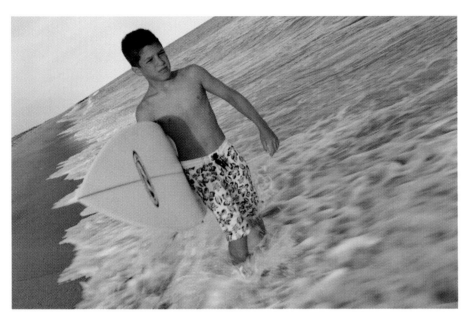

Surfing

- Forward Bend
- Swimmer's Stretch
- Half Moon

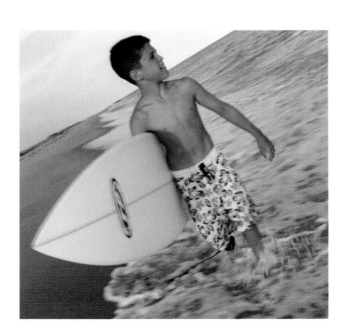

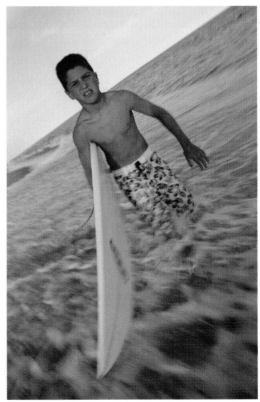

- **Surfers' Back Bend** – Stand with your back to the surfboard and reach over your head to hold the top of the board. Take three full breaths. Arch your back and stretch your chest further with each breath.

  Benefit: stretches and strengthens the torso and encourages full breathing.

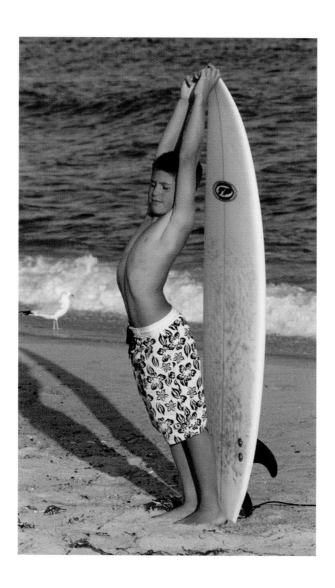

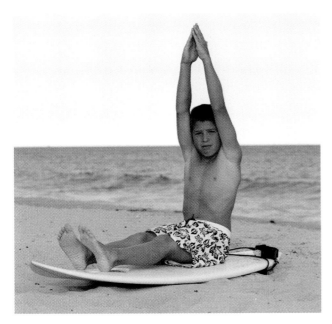

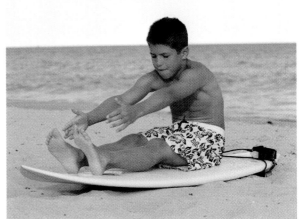

- **Wave Stretch** – Sit on your surf board and inhale as you reach up to the sky. Exhale as you stretch forward over your legs. Reach for your shins, ankles or toes and drop your head. Take two full breaths, stretching further each time.

  Benefit: relieves tension in the lower back and stretches the thighs and calves.

- **Lifeguard Lunge** - Place your surfboard in front of you with its tip dug into the ground. Bend your left knee and stretch the back of your right leg, pressing your right heel into the sand. Hold for a count of three breaths and switch sides.

Benefit: strengthens the thigh and calf muscles and stretches the Achilles tendon.

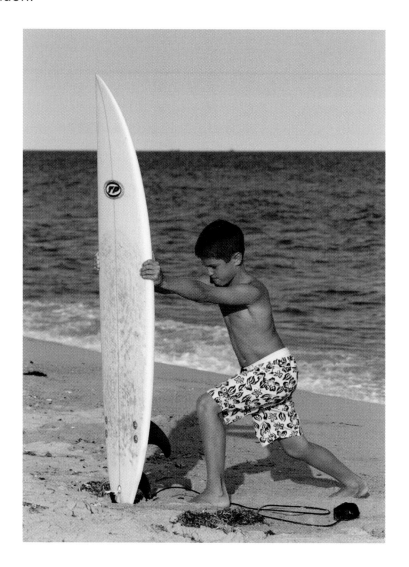

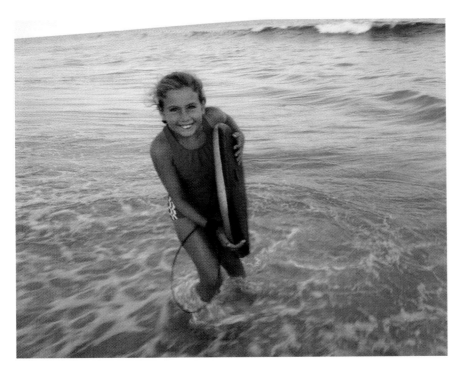

Boogie Boarding

- Forward Bend
- Swimmer's Stretch
- Half Moon

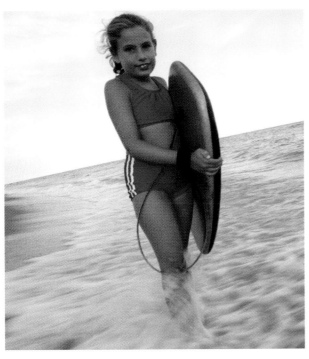

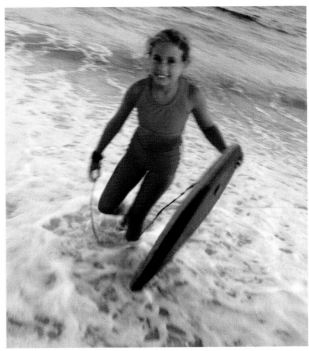

- **Boogie Board Side Stretch** – Hold on to the boogie board and reach it up in the air over your head. Stretch to the right side and take a full breath. Then repeat over the left side.

  Benefit: tones and stretches the torso, and is a good relaxation pose.

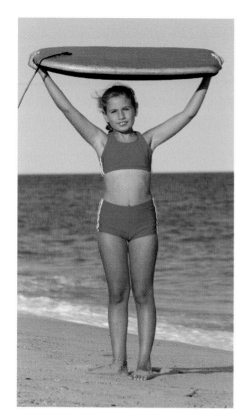
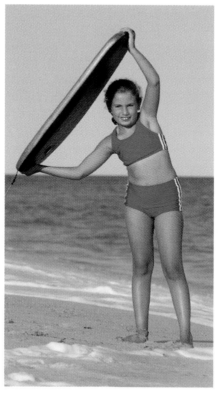
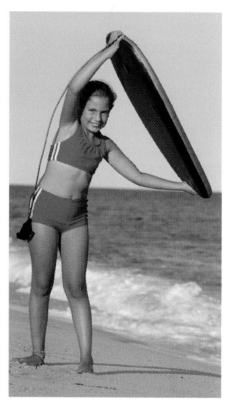

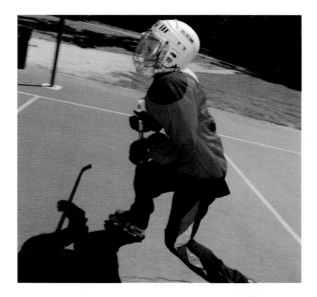

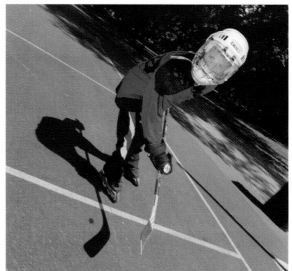

Hockey

- Hurdler
- Bridge
- Butterfly
- Plow

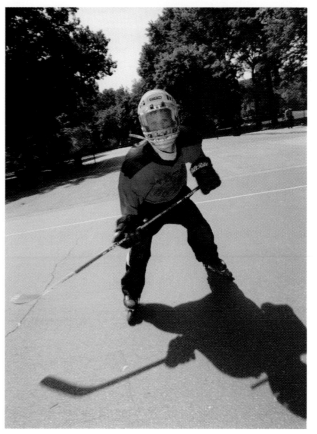

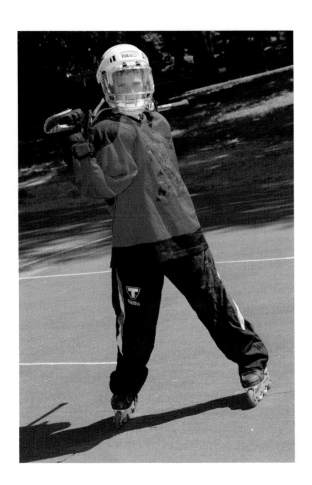 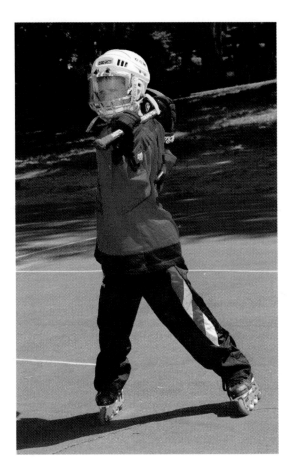

- **Hockey Stick Twist** – Hold the stick behind your head across your shoulders. Keep your lower body still and twist your shoulders to the left. Breathe and twist to the right. Let your head move with your torso.

Benefit: warms up the back and loosens tight muscles.

- **Hat Trick Stretch** – Holding both ends of a hockey stick, reach your arms over your head. Inhale and lower your back, arms and head toward the floor. Exhale and repeat three times.

Benefit: stretches and releases tension in the upper and middle back.

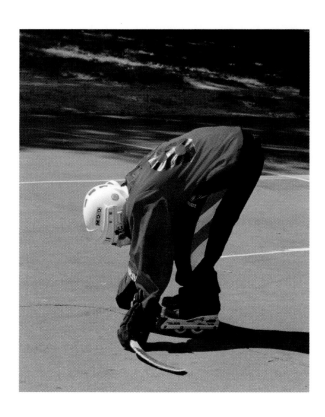
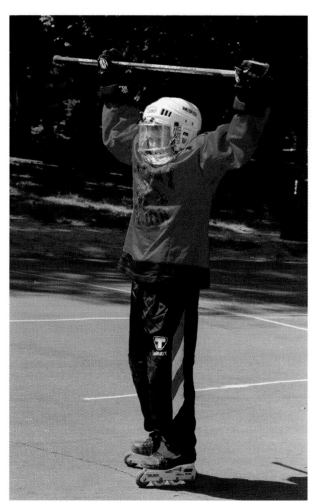

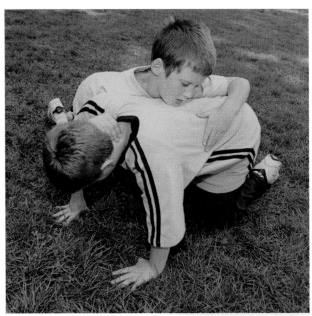

Wrestling

- Straddle
- Hurdler
- Lunge

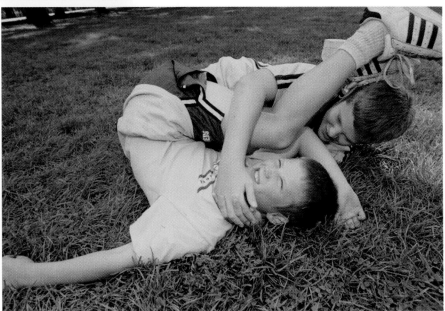

• **Eye of the Needle** – Start on the ground in the cat pose. Reach your right arm to the sky and then down under your torso on the ground. Relax your head and rest on your right shoulder and upper arm as you lift your left arm to the sky. Take three breaths and repeat on the other side.

Benefit: gently stretches the upper back and relieves lower back tension.

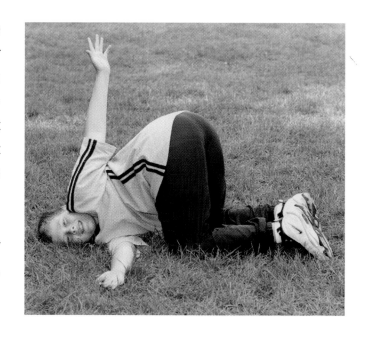

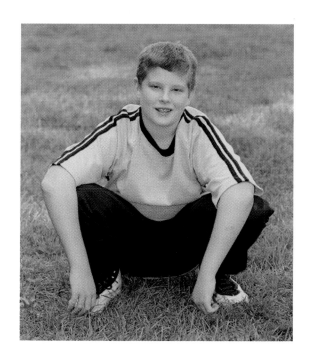

• **Wrestling Squat** – Stand with your feet a little wider then hips-width apart. Keep your knees over your feet and squat until your hips are down to the ground. Hold for three breaths, drop your head and slowly roll up.

Benefit: releases lower back tightness and warms up hips, knees and ankles.

PART VI
DOUBLE YOGA

A great way to share what you have learned practicing yoga is to perform double yoga stretches with your friends. Double yoga is fun and can be a great way to relate to a friend in a new and creative way. While stretching with someone else, you learn to be sensitive to his or her needs. You may take the poses a little further and stretch beyond where you are accustomed to with the help of a

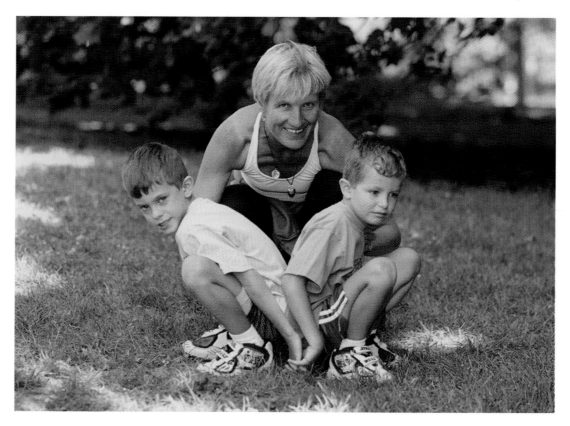

friend. While working with another person, a child might find it easier to concentrate and hold certain positions. Double yoga helps you center yourself while tuning in to your partner.

Double yoga is an exciting new development in the ancient art of yoga. While practicing yoga with another person, you are able to pull against your partner to stretch further and develop strength in the poses. There is often a feeling of invigoration from tuning in to the rhythm of another person. When two people hold a pose together, each partner experiences more energy then he or she contributes.

Subtle lessons in relationships are demonstrated and taught through double yoga. Each child learns to give and take, while communicating mostly non-verbally. Some verbal communication is always encouraged, especially while learning the positions.

Kids learn to literally bend over backwards to assist one another, while remaining centered and focused themselves. Double yoga gives children the opportunity to teach and help someone else. Whether a child practices with a friend or meets someone new, double yoga opens the door to friendship and fun.

Triangle – The triangle pose is the basis of many yoga positions. Start by standing back to back against your partner with your feet spread two to three feet apart. If the two of you are a different height, keep your front feet together and adjust your back leg. Your front feet should be together side to side, while your back feet should be together heel to heel. Keep your legs straight as you reach to your partner's front ankle. Stretch your opposite arm up to the sky and clasp hands. Increase your extension and try to bend from your hips, not your ribs. Be sure to keep your hips facing forward. Switch sides and repeat.

Benefit: great overall body stretch.

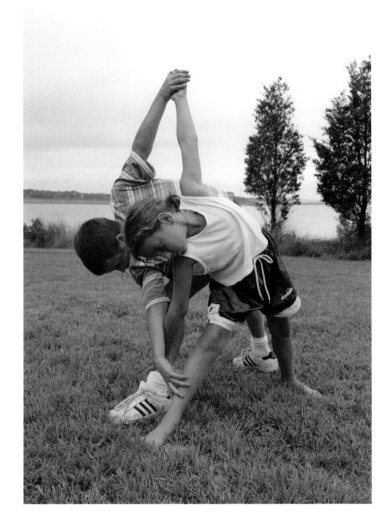

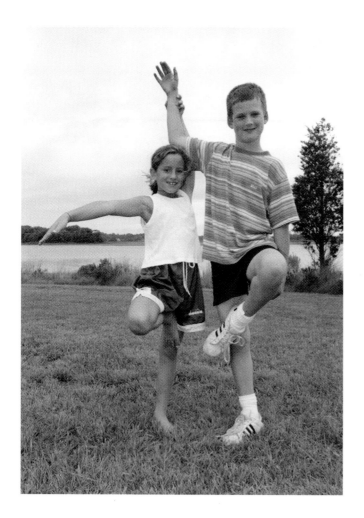

Tree Pose - Stand next to one another and clasp your partner's hand up in the air. Lift your outside foot and rest it against your inner thigh. Rest your outer arm on your bent leg or out to the side for balance. Stand up as straight as possible and try not to lean on your partner. Lift your chest and keep your tailbone down as you focus on a point in front of you. Hold the pose for five full breaths and repeat on the other side.

Benefit: teaches attentive stillness and strengthens the leg muscles.

The Royal Crown – Stand two to three feet apart and face one another. Clasp your hands behind your back. Lean forward, lifting your arms in the air to meet your partner's hands. Take five full breaths.

Benefit: stretches your back, hips and hamstrings.

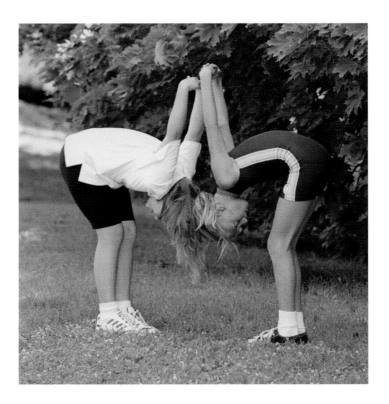

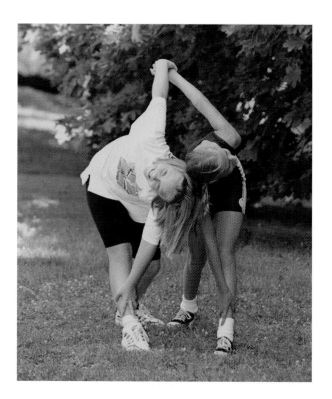

Twisted Triangle – Facing your partner, stand about eight inches apart. From the triangle pose, bend forward from the hips and bring one arm across to your opposite shin. Lift your other arm above your head and hold your partner's hand. Twist your body and press your shoulders together. Breathe and hold for a count of five breaths. Repeat on the other side.

Benefit: stretches the leg muscles, opens the chest and shoulders, relieves tightness, and increases flexibility in the spine.

Hero – Stand next to one another with the sides of your feet together and your opposite foot turned outward. Clasp wrists as you bend your knee and stretch your arm out to the side. Be sure to keep your wrists over the ankles and gently pull away from one another. Repeat on the other side.

Benefit: strengthens the thighs, stretches the hips, and improves posture.

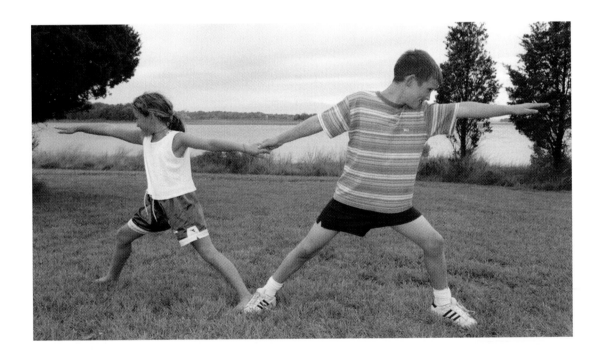

Suspension Bridge – Face your partner standing two to three feet apart. With your feet together and your legs straight, bend from the hips and clasp your partner's hands. Pull your hips back as you extend your spine forward.

Benefit: relieves pressure and tension along the spine, stretches the vertebra, and relieves tension in the back, hips and hamstrings.

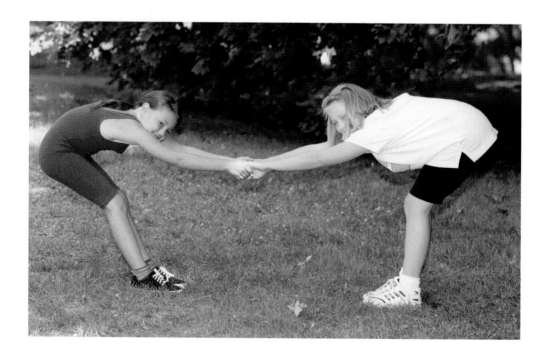

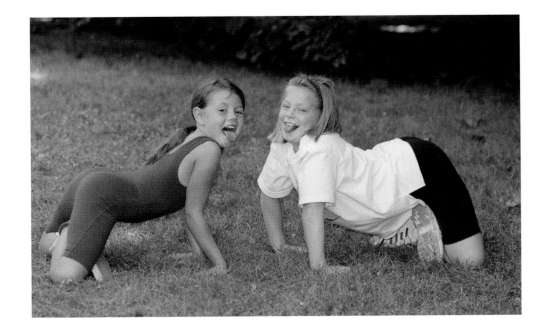

Lotus Lion – Sit in the lotus or half lotus position about four feet apart. Sit up on your knees with your hands on the ground and your fingertips pointing back. Support your torso as you let your hips sink down. Open your mouth as you inhale and exhale.

Benefit: opens the pelvis and increases energy.

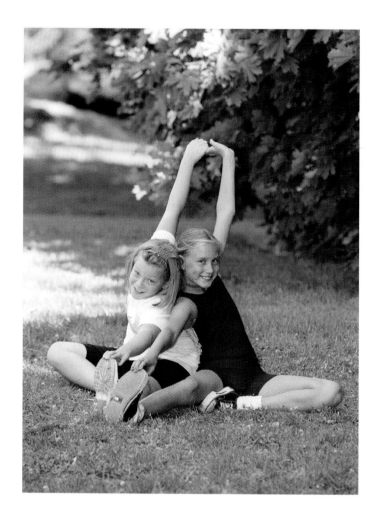

Shooting Star - Sit side by side with the your legs straight and hips touching. Keep your inside leg straight as you place your outside foot against your inner thigh. Reach toward your straight leg, lift your back arm over your head, and hold your partner's hand. Hold the stretch for as long as you can, switch sides and repeat.

Benefit: loosens the hip sockets, stretches the inner thigh and tones the waist.

Cross Gate – Kneel side to side about six feet apart. Extend your inside leg and press the outer edge of your foot against the side of your partner's foot. Hold hands and lean sideways toward each other. Stretch your outside arm over your head and clasp your partner's hand. Hold for a count of five breaths and change sides.

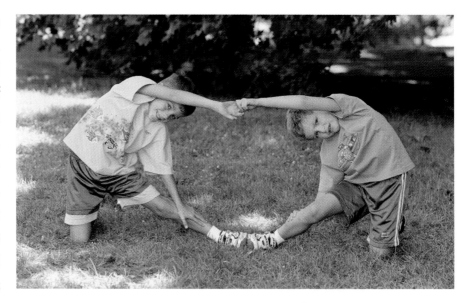

Benefit: this is an intense lateral stretch that removes stiffness from the back and shoulders.

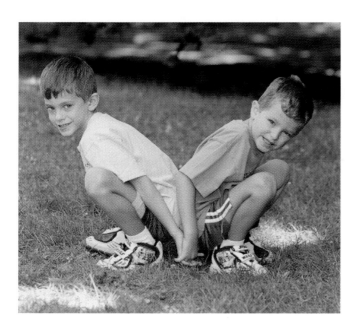

Frog Link – Squat back to back with your feet together and your heels pressed against your partner's. Spread your knees and sink your torso between your thighs. Reach back and clasp your partner's hands. Pull against your partner to feel the stretch from your tailbone to your head.

Benefit: stretches the Achilles tendon and inner thigh.

Straddle – Sit on the ground facing your partner with your legs as far apart as you can stretch. Hold hands and gently pull backward and forward.

Benefit: this pose stretches the inner thighs and pelvis.

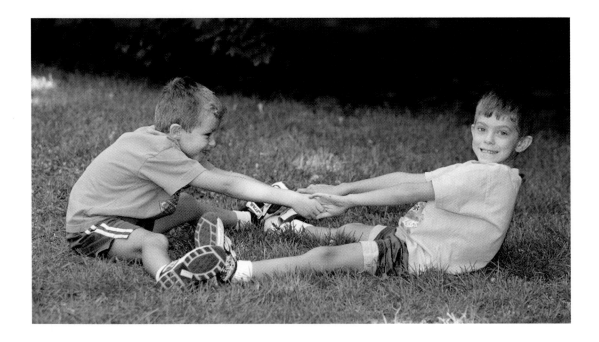

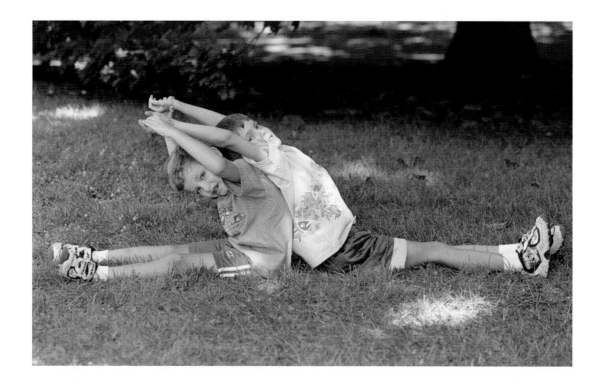

Reclining Forward Bend – Sit back to back with your partner. Keep your legs and arms straight as you hold hands above your head. As your partner performs a forward fold, recline back and feel the stretch in your arms, back and chest. Hold this position for a count of five breaths. Return to center and slowly roll forward, stretching your partner.

Benefit: reclining partner gently stretches the rib muscles, shoulders and armpits, while the folding partner relaxes the back and promotes deep relaxation.

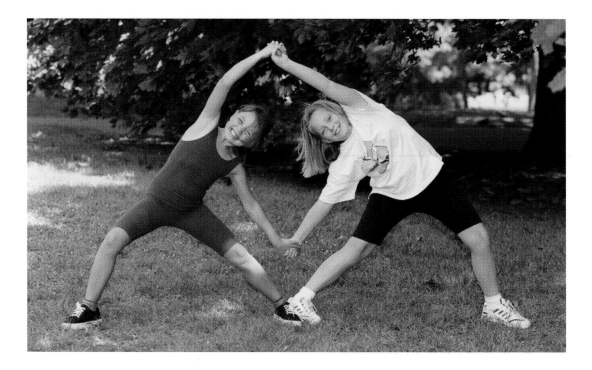

Warrior Diamond – Standing next to one another, start in the warrior pose with your inner feet side to side and hold hands. Reach your outside arms over your head and hold hands above you. Take three long breaths and switch sides.

Benefit: strengthens the thighs and stretches the entire side of the torso.

The Fountain – Stand facing one another with your toes together. Clasp your partner's wrists and lean back. Straighten your elbows and tighten your hips as you maintain an even pull with your partner. Communicate with each other about how far you can each bend back. Lift your chest as you hold the pose and breathe evenly. Repeat three times.

Benefit: lengthens the front of the body and corrects rounded shoulders.

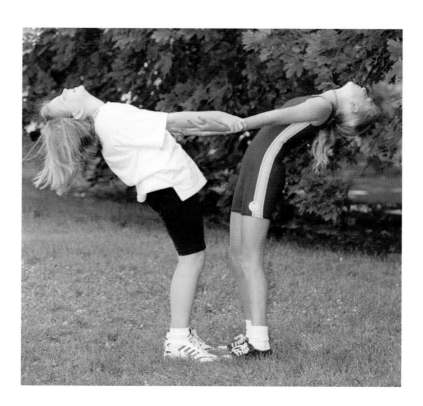

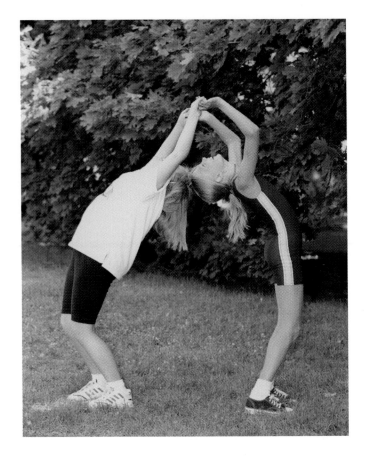

The Arch – Stand about two to three feet apart back to back. Lean backward until the top of your heads touch. Reach overhead and clasp hands. Drop your tailbone and tighten your buttocks. Arch your back and take three long breaths before slowly coming out of the pose.

Benefit: increases circulation up the front of the body and strengthens the back and butt muscles.

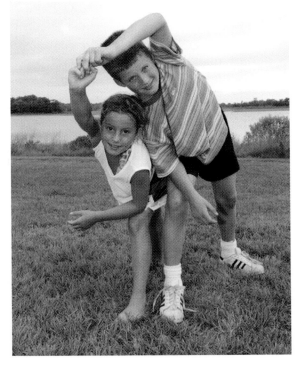

Warrior Side Stretch – Stand back to back in the warrior pose. Lean your forearm on your bent knee and stretch the other arm over your head close to your ear. Hold the pose as you take three full breaths.

Benefit: strengthens the thigh muscles, stretches the torso and encourages full breathing and sensitivity to your partner.

PART VII
YOGA GAMES

An exciting way to vary your yoga routine is to incorporate yoga into some of your favorite outdoor games. Games such as Tag, Twister and Red Light, Green Light can take on another dimension when yoga is added to the fun. Whether they play in a gym, in the back yard or at the park, kids get all the benefits of yoga–stretching, twisting, and balancing–while exploring different positions. Games get children of all different ages and fitness levels together. Some children are athletic while others are not, but all kids can have a lot of fun playing yoga games.

Twister

Find your old twister game and play with as few as two or as many as four people. As you play the game, see how many yoga or yoga-like poses you can get into as you move your hands and feet around the mat. If you find yourself in an unusual position, take it to its maximum stretch and

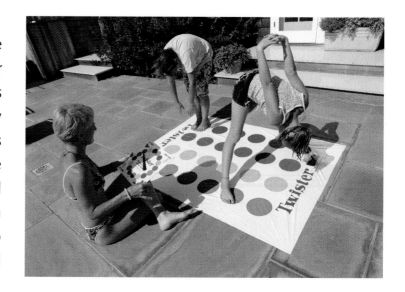

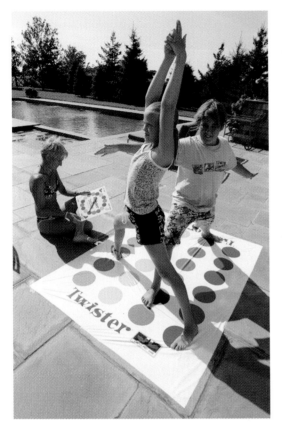

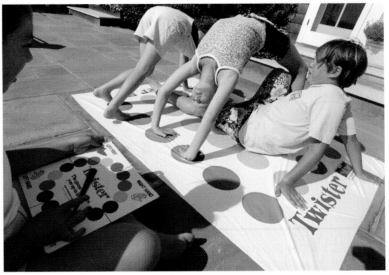

breathe. Intertwine yourself in your friend's yoga poses. In between your turns, practice three-part breathing while holding the twister position.

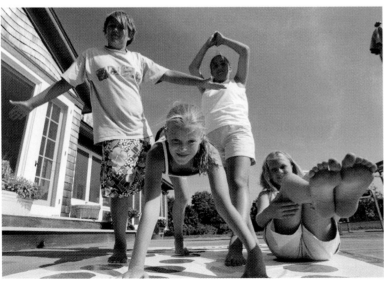

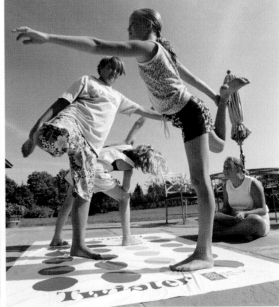

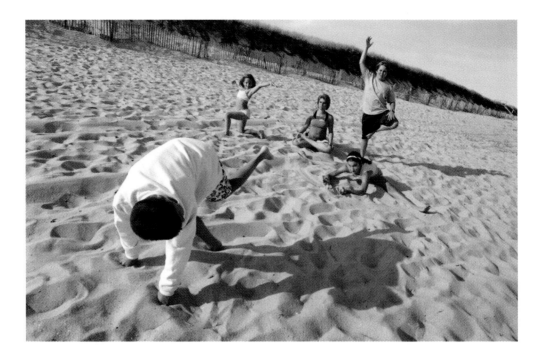

Red Light Green Light, 1, 2, 3

This game is usually played outside on a lawn or at the beach. All the kids line up and one person stands a few feet in front of them. The child in front calls out "red light, green light, 1, 2, 3" and turns around. All the kids run forward to-

ward the caller. When she turns around, everyone freezes in a yoga pose. If someone is spotted moving, they have to go back to the starting line. The first person to reach the caller is "it." Remember to breathe and be imaginative. Try to get into different poses each time you freeze.

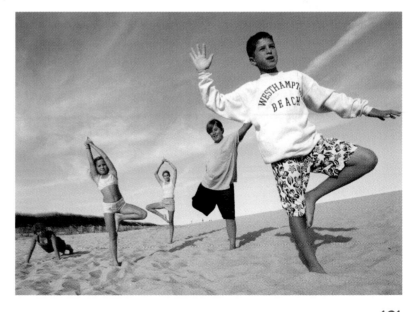

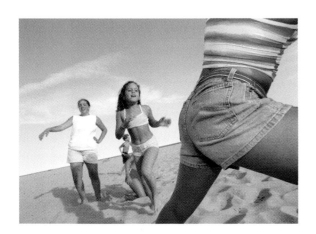

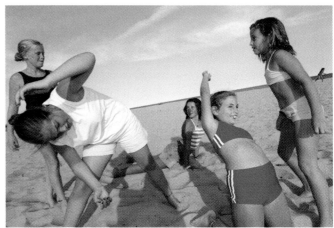

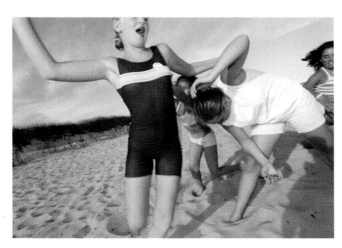

Freeze Tag

A great game to play outdoors, one person is "it" and everyone runs around. When the person who is "it" tags someone, they freeze into a yoga pose until a team member frees them by climbing over or crawling under them.

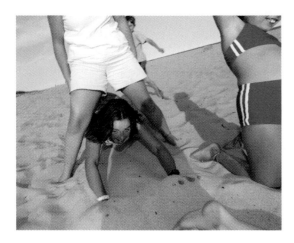

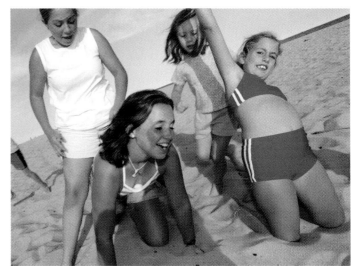

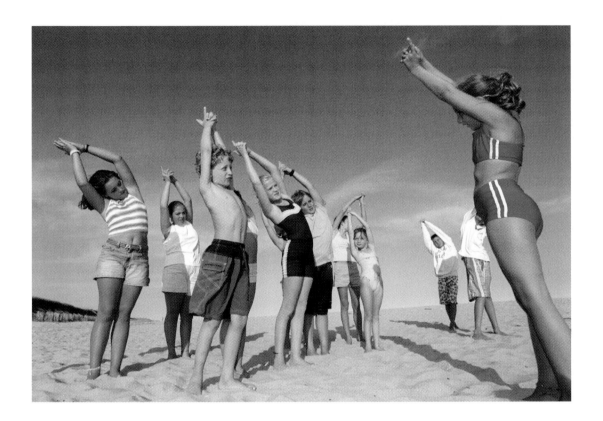

Simon Says

The leader calls out yoga poses by saying "Simon says get in the tree pose," and everyone follows. If the leader calls out a yoga poses without starting the sentence with "Simon says," anyone who follows is out (example: "Get in the tree pose"). The last one to remain in the game is the next leader.

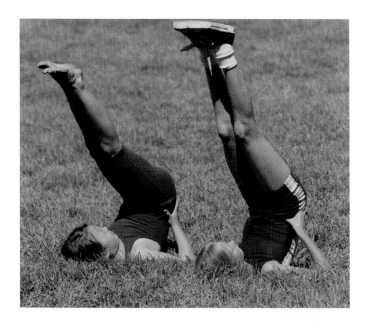

Shadow Yoga

Partner up with someone else. One person does a yoga pose as the other one performs the mirror image of the pose. Each person should do five poses with the partner mirroring, then switch.

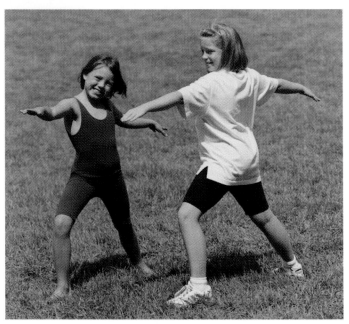

PART VIII
SALUTATIONS

Salutations were named after the sun and the moon because they are especially good to do first thing in the morning to wake up or last thing at night to cool down. In the morning, I suggest warming up into salutations slowly, then increasing the tempo and intensity. In the evenings, do three salutations slowly and remember to breathe fully. This will prepare you for a sound sleep and sweet dreams. There has been a connection found between going to sleep relaxed and remembering your dreams.

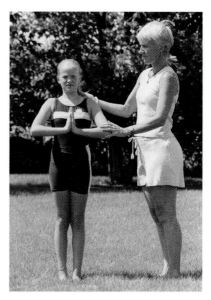

Sun Salutations are perfectly balanced yoga sequences. Salutations are very efficient, reaching almost every major muscle group in the body. Salutations flow from one yoga posture to the next, connected by breathing. It is important to breathe fully and not to hold your breath. We naturally have a tendency to hold our breath when learning something new. Knowing when to inhale and exhale will come naturally with practice. The salutations are balanced workouts because they combine forward bending, backward bending, stretching side to side and twisting.

SALUTATION #1

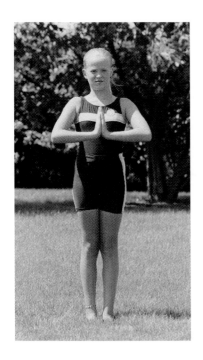

1. Prayer

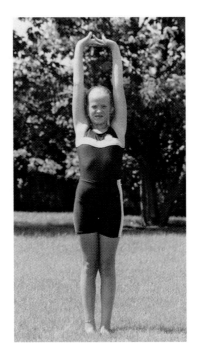

2. Mountain
Variation

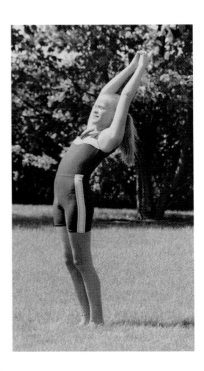

3. Half Moon
Backbend

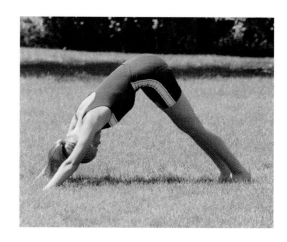

6. Down Dog

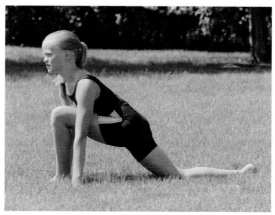

5. Lunge, right leg back

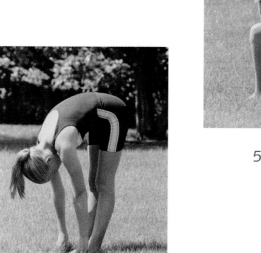

4. Forward Fold

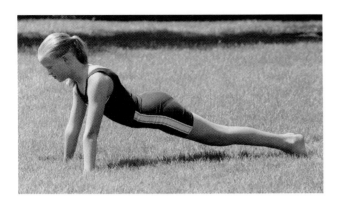

7. Plank

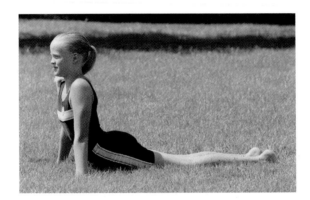

8. Up Dog

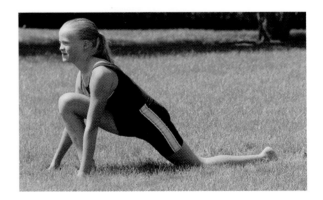

9. Lunge, left leg back

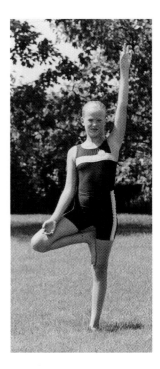

13. Tree

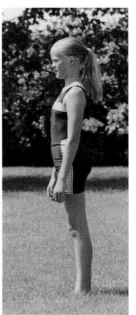

12. Mountain
Variation

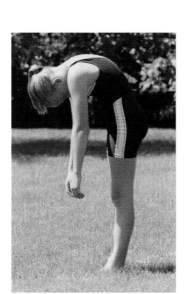

11. Roll Up

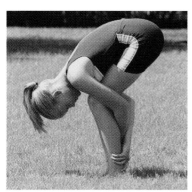

10. Forward Bend

SALUTATIONS #2

1. Mountain
2. Half Moon
3. Forward Bend
4. Lunge, left leg back
5. Warrior, right leg bent
6. Triangle Spinal Twist, left hand to right leg
7. Down Dog
8. Plank
9. Up Dog
10. Lunge, right leg back
11. Warrior, left leg bent
12. Triangle Spinal Twist, right hand to left leg
13. Swimmer's Stretch
14. Mountain

SALUTATIONS #3

1. Mountain
2. Swimmer's Stretch
3. Lunge, right leg back
4. Triangle Side Stretch, stretch to the left
5. Down Dog
6. Cat Pose
7. Child Pose
8. Cobra
9. Down Dog
10. Lunge, left leg back
11. Triangle Side Stretch, stretch to the right
12. Forward Fold
13. Mountain

PART IX
YOGA ROUTINES

Headache Eraser
Half Lotus
Seated Side Stretch
Eye Relaxation
  – Brow and Lids
Shoulder Self-Massage
Neck Rolls

Morning Wake-Up
Angel Breath
Child Pose
Butterfly
Half Bridge
Cat
Down Dog
Sun Salutation #1
Sun Salutation #2

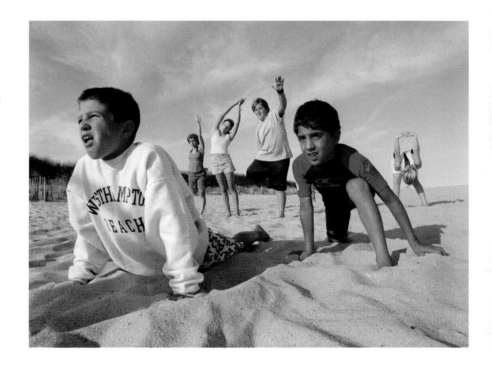

Studying Stress Reducer
Mountain Pose
Half Moon*
Forward Bend*
Swimmer's Stretch
Fire Breath
Shoulder Rolls
Neck Rolls
Shoulder Self-Massage
(* can also be done seated)

Sweet Dreams
Sun Salutation #3
Half Moon
Child Pose
Camel
Straddle
Hurdler
Half Bridge
Plow
Shoulder Stand
Fish

Test Centering
Cross-Legged Position
Three-Part Breath
Angel Breaths
Eye Relaxation – Lid, Brow, and Clock
Neck Rolls
Shoulder Rolls
Shoulder Self-Massage

PART X
RELAXATION

We all need to learn basic relaxation techniques to help us in our everyday lives. If taught at a young age, these techniques will always remain in a child's muscle memory. Here is a simple guided relaxation that can be read out loud to kids in a group or individually. A child can read it to a friend, or a parent can read it to a child. The relaxation should be done in a quiet place with few distractions.

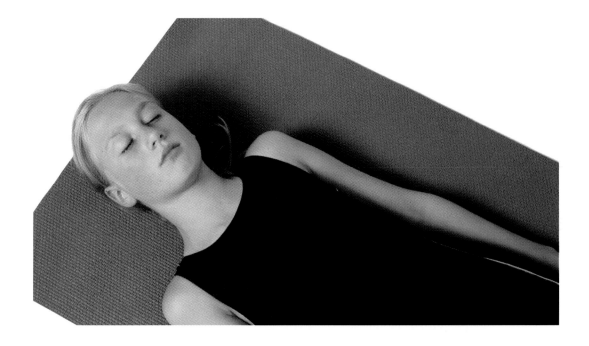

Lie on your back. Tighten all the muscles in your body and then release them. Then tighten all the muscles on the right side of your body–your face, arm, hand, hip, leg, and foot–and release. Then, tighten all the muscles on the left side of your body and release. Close your eyes and feel your body sink into the floor. For the next few minutes, focus on how your body is feeling and notice how you are breathing. Feel your stomach lift as you inhale and lower as you exhale. Count five slow breaths, relaxing more with each exhale.

Follow my voice as we travel through the body to release tension, tightness and worry. Feel the back of your head relax against the ground. Let go of any fixed expression on your face. Relax the muscles around your eyes, jaw and mouth. Feel your neck release in the front, sides and back. Let go of your upper back, shoulders and chest. If you feel tension or get distracted, take a deep breath and focus on relaxing your muscles. Notice your chest expand as you inhale, filling your lungs with air.

Feel tightness and tension leave your body as you exhale. Breathe easily as you feel your stomach rise as you inhale and lower as you exhale. Take a few deep breaths. With each inhale, feel cool fresh air enter and fill your lungs. As you exhale, feel the air that has been warmed by your body exit through your nose and mouth. Feel your middle back release into the ground and the weight of your hips and legs sink into gravity. Notice your right leg, knee and foot release. Notice the left leg, knee and foot let go.

Imagine a wave of relaxation travel over the front of your body from your toes up your legs to your hips, and across your stomach, chest, neck and face. Feel this wave erase any tightness or worry from your mind and body. Feel the wave of relaxation travel from the top of your head to the heels of your feet. Now inhale slowly and feel the circulation travel up the front of your body. Exhale as you feel it travel down the back of your body. Notice this light, relaxed,

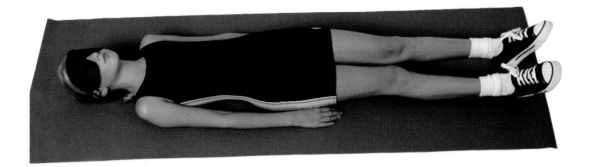

centered feeling. Open your eyes. Roll to the right side and slowly sit up into a cross-legged position.

Test-Centering Relaxation

This is a great technique for students to do on their own or for teachers to read to their classes. This relaxation is especially helpful the morning of a test day. Sit cross-legged or in a chair. Close your eyes, relax your facial muscles and drop your shoulders. Tune into the cool air coming in through your nose. Hold the air in your lungs for a few moments before slowly exhaling. Repeat and inhale for a count of three, hold, and exhale for a count of three. Relax and clear your mind. Focus on breathing as you fill yourself with confidence and clarity. Open your eyes and feel refreshed.

Travel Relaxation

Whether you are in a car, bus or plane, it is a perfect time to practice a relaxation. Take your shoes off and rotate your ankles three times in each direction. Flex and point your feet three times. Roll down your spine and slowly roll back up. Arch and round the spine, inhaling as you arch and exhaling as you round your back three times. Do three shoulder rolls and a seated spinal twist to the left. Gain leverage with your left arm over the back of your seat and gaze over your left shoulder. Take a deep breath and repeat on the other side. Return facing forward and close your eyes. Feel a wave of relaxation travel up and down your spine. Imagine traveling to a beautiful and relaxing place. Think of what you might see, hear and feel in this paradise. Picture this place clearly in your mind's eye. Allow yourself to drift off in your imagination. As you come out of your relaxation, start to wiggle your toes. Feel the circulation spiral up your body and open your eyes. You should feel alert but relaxed.

PART XI
A FINAL NOTE

After many years of teaching yoga to adults, expanding my classes to include children was a natural progression. Yoga can be so beneficial and fun for kids to do. In my yoga classes for children, kids are always surprised that something that is so enjoyable can make them feel so good afterwards.

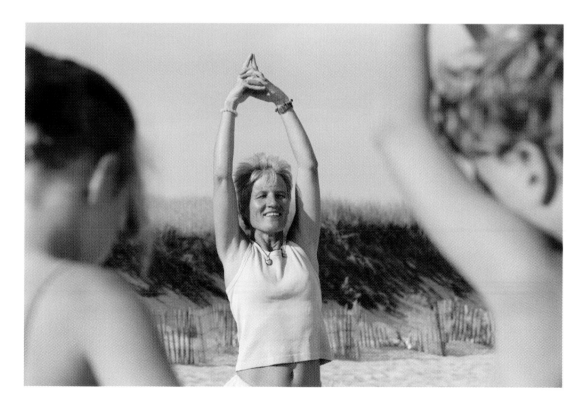

Yoga taps into kids' imagination and feeds their curiosity. They love hearing about the history of yoga and about poses they can do alone or with friends. Kids love learning about the fun names of yoga exercises and often enjoy naming or re-naming the poses themselves.

Whether kids want to relax, play games or participate in sports, yoga can be a valuable addition to their lives. It's a great skill to share with other kids, parents and teachers. As a full yoga workout or a stretching routine before an athletic event, kids can use I Can't Believe It's Yoga for Kids to best fit their lifestyles. Start practicing yoga now and you'll be on your way to a lifetime of better mental and physical health.

Lisa Trivell

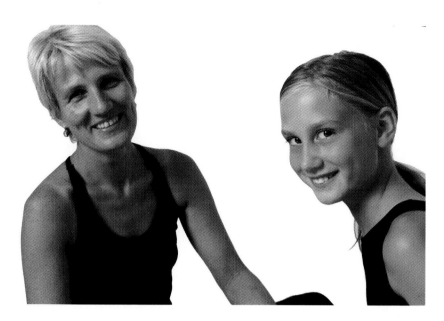

Lisa Trivell with her daughter Amanda.

Meet the Author

Lisa Trivell is a certified exercise and yoga instructor, as well as a licensed massage therapist. For 15 years, she has taught yoga in New York City and East Hampton in corporations, schools, and her private practice. She is certified by the International Fitness Professionals Association (IFPA) and the American Aerobics Association International / International Sports Medicine Association (AAAI / ISMA).

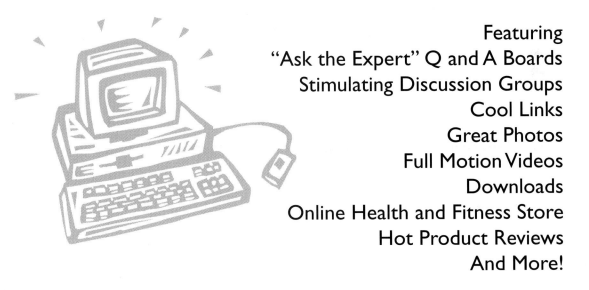

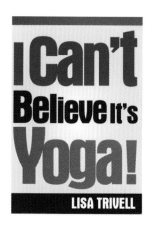

I Can't Believe It's Yoga!

It's Yoga — American Style

Lisa Trivell, Photographed by Peter Field Peck

A popular form of exercise and fitness conditioning, yoga combines stretching and breathing to tone the body, relax the muscles, and relieve tension. The numerous benefits of yoga can easily be added to anyone's daily fitness routine.

For many, though, yoga is seen as being both too difficult and too different to try. *I Can't Believe It's Yoga* addresses this perception problem by presenting a yoga based fitness program which is easy to accomplish.

In *I Can't Believe It's Yoga*, Lisa Trivell, an experienced yoga instructor transforms even the reluctant skeptic into an avid fan. Utilizing the most basic yoga exercises, the results are incredible!

IBSN 1-57826-032-9 / $14.95

**Available in bookstores everywhere,
order toll free
at 1-800-906-1234
or online at getfitnow.com.**

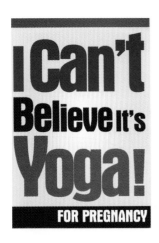